Heal
Pelvic
Pain

A Proven Stretching, Strengthening, and Nutrition Program for Relieving Pain, Incontinence, IBS, and Other Symptoms *Without Surgery*

Heal

Pelvic

Pain

AMY STEIN, M.P.T.

FOREWORD BY ANDREW GOLDSTEIN, M.D.

New York   Chicago   San Francisco   Lisbon   London   Madrid   Mexico City
Milan   New Delhi   San Juan   Seoul   Singapore   Sydney   Toronto

The *McGraw·Hill* Companies

Library of Congress Cataloging-in-Publication Data

Stein, Amy.
    Heal pelvic pain : the proven stretching, strengthening, and nutrition program
for relieving pain, incontinence, IBS, and other symptoms without surgery /
by Amy Stein.
        p.   cm.
    Includes index.
    ISBN 978-0-07-154656-0 (alk. paper)
    MHID   0-07-154656-1 (alk. paper)
    1. Pelvic floor—Diseases—Exercise therapy.   2. Pelvic floor—Diseases—Physical
therapy.   I. Title.

RC946.S74   2009
616.7'10642—dc22   2008002072

2 3 4 5 6 7 8 9 10 11 12 13 14 15 16 17 18 19 20 21   DOC/DOC 0 9

ISBN 978-0-07-154656-0
MHID   0-07-154656-1

Interior photographs copyright © Richard Hutchings
Illustrations by Marie Dauenheimer

McGraw-Hill books are available at special quantity discounts to use as premiums and
sales promotions or for use in corporate training programs. To contact a representative,
please visit the Contact Us pages at www.mhprofessional.com.

This book is printed on acid-free paper.

CONTENTS

FOREWORD

When I was in medical school back in the 1990s, physical therapy (PT) was regarded as something of an afterthought. Since physical therapists rarely published studies in journals read by physicians, the PT practice lacked scientific clout—at least as far as doctors were concerned. When physical therapy *was* considered, it was seen as useful mostly for damaged muscles and joints after injury or surgery. In other words, after doctors had done the real work, you might prescribe physical therapy for the mop-up.

Despite completing nearly 20,000 hours of internship and residency in obstetrics and gynecology, I heard only one hour-long lecture on vulvar pain and sexual dysfunction. I was taught that pain during sex was the result of "vaginismus," an involuntary contraction of the vaginal muscles during attempted penetration. I was further taught that vaginismus was a psychological issue resulting from trauma or abuse, and that it was to be treated through psychotherapy and sex therapy. Physical therapy was never mentioned. Other types of vulvar pain were thought to be caused by nerve injury and were treated—as much as possible—with drugs. Again, physical therapy was never discussed as a treatment for women suffering this pain, nor was I ever taught anything about pelvic floor disorders in men!

After completing my residency, I joined the faculty of Johns Hopkins and became the director for the Center for Vulvovaginal Disorders. A great many of the patients with whom I dealt had suffered pain for a decade or more. Prescription drugs controlled the pain, but they did not cure it and often produced significant side effects—including heart palpitations, extreme lethargy, weight gain, dry mouth, and constipation. If it was a steep price for these women to pay for the relief of their pain, few people in the medical profession questioned the situation or challenged the assumptions on which this standard therapy was based—namely, that the chronic pain was solely due to nerve injury—neuropathy, in medical lingo.

The only problem with this "wisdom" was that it wasn't true. It took some forward-looking physical therapists like Amy Stein, the very folks we doctors had typically paid little attention to, to enlighten us on what was really at issue.

It's not too far-fetched to say that Amy and her colleagues had to beat down the doors of the medical establishment—figuratively, anyway—to be heard. They made their case with compelling logic, arguing that the cause of much of the pain we were treating with medication was not, in fact, neuropathic, but instead myofascial—that is, in the muscles and tissue. The pain, they explained, was a result of the muscles having tightened and shortened. The tightening had decreased the blood flow and therefore the supply of oxygen to the affected muscles; as a result, lactic acid built up, irritating the nerves that pass through the muscles. As the brain perceives pain as being located in the end organ reached by the affected nerve, the person felt vulvar pain. In addition, the irritation of the nerve typically gives rise to an inflammation that produces redness and swelling, and the redness and swelling, like the pain, show up in the "endpoint" organ reached by the irritated nerve—namely, the vulva.

Examining patients presenting with a complaint of pain in the vulva and with redness and swelling visible in the vulva, doctors would typically diagnose a vulvar infection, prescribing treatment that patients did not need for infections they did not have—treatments that were often irritating and sometimes harmful. Similarly, doctors often diagnosed prostatitis in men when the real issue was a pelvic floor disorder that could be addressed without drugs and without surgery.

As compelling as the arguments of these farsighted physical therapists were, what was really convincing was to see the profound and stunning results that Amy and the other physical therapists achieved when I began referring patients to them. I can describe those results in one simple but powerful word: cure. Through the modalities of physical therapy—manipulation, massage, and above all exercises that patients could do on their own—women who had suffered "chronic" pain for years stopped suffering.

This wasn't just temporary relief from pain. It wasn't a palliative. It was a cure. The women were able to give up the medications that had been controlling their pain, and they were able to return to normal functioning in every way—just by learning to relax and let go of the tension in their muscles, learning to lengthen their muscles, and learning to strengthen their muscles in the right way.

The impact on my practice of finding this natural cure has been phenomenal. I estimate that today I refer at least 50 percent of my patients to Amy Stein and other physical therapists who specialize in the disorders of the pelvic floor. I could not be a vulvar specialist without their very important specialty.

Many of the pain syndromes doctors and patients have struggled with for years now turn out to derive from myofascial disorders. For example, women are frequently diagnosed with irritable bowel syndrome or interstitial cystitis when in fact all of their pain may be myofascial in origin.

We live in a somewhat puritanical society, where the issues of pelvic floor disorder are not discussed openly, if at all. What's more, our culture's attitude toward health care often encourages the quick fix—make an appointment and get a prescription—and certainly, our current system of health-care insurance favors such efficiency. In France, however, it has long been the custom for every woman who goes through a vaginal delivery to see a physical therapist as part of her postpartum treatment. The muscles are massaged, lengthened, stretched, and strengthened prophylactically so as to prevent the weakness that can lead to incontinence or the tightness that can result from a tear or episiotomy and can lead to so much pain, discomfort, and limitations on functioning.

We also tend to believe that there's so much health-care information available—in newspapers and magazines and all over the Internet—that we should be in charge of our own medical treatment, even to the point of self-diagnosis and self-medication. Studies show, however, that when a woman diagnoses herself with a yeast infection based on the symptoms of itching, burning, and discharge—to take a common example—she is incorrect more than 50 percent of the time. The symptoms are just as likely to be a result of nerve irritation or tightened tissue. Yet far too many women head to the drugstore for creams to treat chronic itching and burning—often with dire consequences—when what they really should be doing is the exercise program in this book.

And that's precisely why this book is so important. It speaks openly and candidly to readers about the pain they are experiencing and the root causes of that pain. And it offers them simple, practical therapies for curing the pain so they can return to fully functioning lives. When the life-limiting pain and discomfort of pelvic floor disorder are at issue, Amy's program of exercises and self-care techniques is absolutely the best medicine.

Andrew T. Goldstein, M.D., FACOG
Director, The Centers for Vulvovaginal Disorders
Washington, D.C., and New York City
Coauthor, *Reclaiming Desire: Four Keys to Finding Your Lost Libido*

ACKNOWLEDGMENTS

My first thank-you is to my patients. They have been my biggest inspiration to learn more and to educate the public on pelvic pain and pelvic floor disorders. In addition, I'm grateful to those doctors and health-care providers who believe in these patients, and who understand the power of physical therapy to cure musculoskeletal pelvic floor disorders.

My agent, Sarah Jane Freymann, was really the progenitor of the idea for this book. I am grateful to her, McGraw-Hill editors Johanna Bowman and Craig Bolt, and copyeditor Alison Shurtz for understanding the importance of the book and for making it happen; to Susanna Margolis for helping get the book out of me; to Amy and Richard Hutchings of Hutchings Photography for the beautiful photos; and to Marie Dauenheimer for the great illustrations.

To everyone at Beyond Basics Physical Therapy who continues to help more than 5,000 sufferers each year, your success and passion are in this book; I couldn't have done it without you.

Finally, I am grateful to my entire support network—my family, my friends, and Travis—for their unconditional love and support.

CHAPTER 1

AT THE BODY'S CORE

Say good-bye to your pelvic pain.

No matter how much it hurts, no matter how long you've suffered, no matter how many different pills you've taken or treatments you've undergone, the program in this book can help alleviate your pain or disorder and start the healing.

No drugs, no surgery. Instead, this is a program of natural healing—of exercises, massage, nutrition, and self-care therapies that will focus on the true underlying condition of your pain. Heal the condition, and your symptoms will go away—and that's just what the program in this book can help you achieve.

To start, I'll explain what pelvic floor disorder is, why doctors have trouble diagnosing it, why you may have had so much trouble treating it so far, and how you can feel better as quickly as possible.

The first thing you should know is that you are not alone. Of course, nobody likes to talk about bladder problems or painful sex or itching or burning in the genital region, so you may not hear or read much about pelvic floor disorders. But the truth is that millions of us suffer from these disorders—women and men, athletes and couch potatoes, young and old, even children.

Mostly, it's women who suffer. As I write this, 9.2 million women have pelvic floor disorder but don't know it because it has not been properly diagnosed. And the sad fact is that if you're a woman, you have at least a 5 percent chance of suffering chronic pelvic pain.

But your pain right now is what counts. That's why you're reading this book. You may be one of the more than 30 million women who have irritable bowel syndrome or one of the 700,000 with the urinary frequency, urgency, and pain that are collectively referred to as painful bladder syndrome or interstitial cystitis.

Maybe you suffer some form of incontinence, especially if you gave birth recently or exercise frequently.

Maybe you have some form of sexual dysfunction; 43 percent of women do. Pain during intercourse, performance problems, and declines in sexual response and enjoyment are all more common than you think. All can adversely affect your relationship with your partner. And all can be treated with the natural healing program in this book.

THE PELVIC FLOOR

What is the pelvic floor? Take a look at the figures. The pelvic floor is all the muscles, plus the nerves controlling the muscles, plus the tissues—called fascia—that connect everything together, plus the ligaments that link bone to bone and bone to organ that are attached to the front, back, and sides of the pelvis, from the pubic bone in the front of the body all the way back to the tailbone. These muscles, nerves, tissues, and ligaments sheathe the floor of the pelvis and together act like a sling or hammock to support the pelvic organs—the urinary tract, digestive tract, and reproductive organs—including the bladder, the uterus (or in men, the prostate), and the colon.

This is an essential part of your body's core, the center of gravity in your frame, the place where movement originates—in a sense, the seat of raw power in your body. Eastern religions attribute spir-

Figure 1.1 Female Urogenital System (midsagittal section)

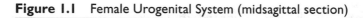

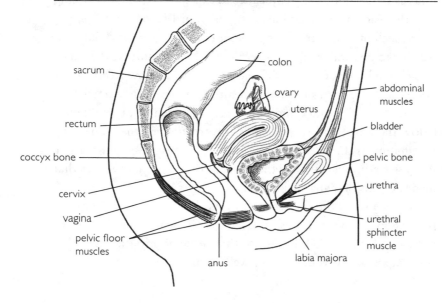

Figure 1.2 Male Urogenital System (midsagittal section)

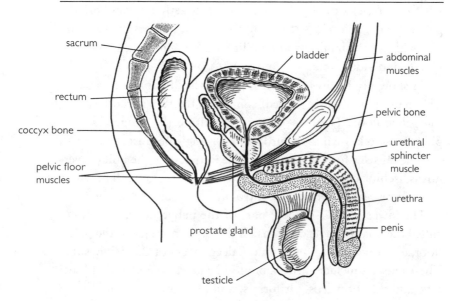

itual as well as physical significance to this part of the body, seeing it as the place where the vital energy of your life force resides.

In much of Hindu tradition, it is the coiled serpent of *Kundalini*, waiting to be awakened into energy. In Chinese culture, the pelvic floor is the home of *chi*, the life energy that must flow freely in our bodies in order for us to remain healthy. In Japanese martial arts, it is the *hara*, the vital center of the self—located just three fingers below the navel and three fingers inward toward the spine. The recognition of this vital life force is at the heart of spiritual practice in these traditions, and it is the focus of the physical exercises that invariably accompany such practices.

Western scientific research confirms that a strong and healthy pelvic floor at the core is essential to overall health and fitness. It's critical to feeling good. It's key to that sense of physical vigor that is so important to your sense of well-being.

THE MUSCLES OF THE PELVIC FLOOR

All the muscles of the pelvic floor work together to support the pelvic organs and to assist in bladder, bowel, and sexual function and with trunk stability and mobility. But each muscle also has its specific individual role.

As shown in Figures 1.3 and 1.4, the pelvic floor has two parts. The upper part (lightly shaded) comprises the superficial layers of the pelvic floor. The muscles here constitute the urogenital diaphragm, also known as the urogenital triangle because, as you can see, the muscles form a triangle. These muscles are the bulbocavernosus, ischiocavernosus, and the transverse perineum, all of which assist in orgasm and bladder control in both men and women.

The lower (darker-shaded) part of the pelvic floor, sometimes called the anal triangle contains all the other muscles of the pelvic floor, all of which are found in the deep layers of the pelvic sling. These muscles include the levator ani, the urethral and anal sphincters, and the coccygeus, piriformis, and obturator internus.

Figure 1.3 Female Pelvic Floor Anatomy

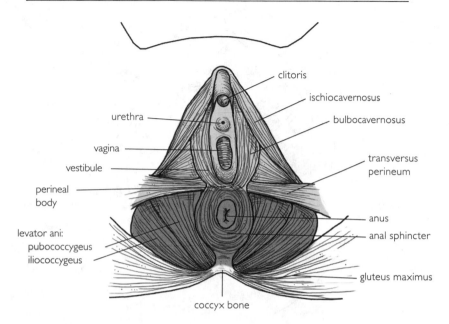

Figure 1.4 Male Pelvic Floor Anatomy

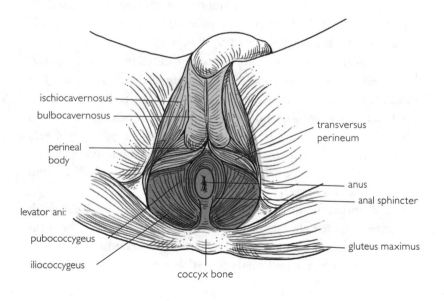

Figure 1.5 Coccygeus, Piriformis, and Obturator Internus

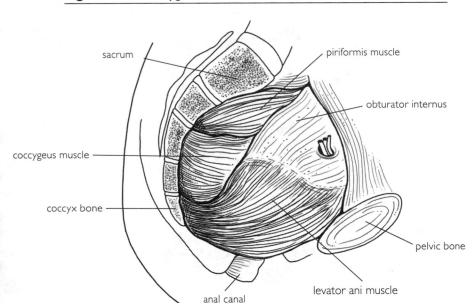

sacrum

piriformis muscle

obturator internus

coccygeus muscle

coccyx bone

pelvic bone

levator ani muscle

anal canal

The levator ani muscle moves the coccyx or tailbone. It is made up of the pubococcygeus (an important muscle that assists in orgasm in men and women), the puborectalis, and the iliococcygeus (see Figures 1.3, 1.4, and 1.5). You won˜t see the puborectalis labeled in the illustrations because it is located beneath the pubococcygeus muscle. Both muscles originate at the pubic bone. The pubococcygeus attaches to the coccyx bone, or tailbone, and the puborectalis wraps around the rectum. The puborectalis assists in bowel emptying; therefore, if the puborectalis is tight or spasmed, this might result in incomplete or difficult bowel emptying.

The urethral and anal sphincter muscles assist in bladder and bowel function in men and women.

The obturator internus, coccygeus, and piriformis all work together but have slightly different roles (see Figure 1.5). The obturator internus is also a hip rotator and is the conduit for a very important nerve, the pudendal nerve, that helps control a great deal of pelvic floor function. A dysfunction in the obturator internus can therefore result in a slew of problems. The coccygeus muscle assists the levator ani muscles in moving the coccyx bone or tailbone when the muscles are contracted. The piriformis, like the obturator internus, is also a hip rotator.

Experts in evolution theorize that the pelvic floor musculature once controlled the tails of our apelike ancestors, before hands proved to be more effective. Eventually, the use of hands naturally selected a new branch of evolutionary development. In that new branch, which eventually became us, the tails went away, but the muscles remained. Now, however, instead of controlling wagging and hanging from trees, the muscles took on the function of helping to support the body's core. So today, the evolved pelvic floor serves three vital purposes:

- It upholds and cushions the organs within the pelvis and lower abdomen: urinary organs, digestive organs, and reproductive organs.
- It controls continence by signaling elimination urges to the bladder and bowel and by opening and closing the urethra and anal canals to allow voiding.
- It is the mechanism of sexual function, contracting the muscles around the female and male genitalia to respond to arousal and to enhance appreciation.

These are big and important jobs, which may be why so many thick, closely connected muscles are involved. We can characterize these pelvic floor muscles in several ways.

First, they're voluntary muscles. That is, we control them consciously. This is different from the smooth muscles of the bladder, intestines, lungs, and blood vessels, which are involuntary; that is, they're controlled by our nervous systems in such a way that they operate automatically.

Second, the muscles of the pelvic floor are skeletal muscles. That means they are attached to the skeletal frame. When we contract the pelvic floor muscles, the energy of the contraction applies force to the tailbone.

The pelvic floor muscles also come in two "speeds." About 70 percent of the pelvic floor muscle fibers are slow-twitch or slow-contraction fibers; the rest are fast-twitch fibers.

Put simply, the slow-twitch muscle fibers fuel endurance. They're the marathoners of muscles, providing support and resisting fatigue. Think of the muscles in your lower back: they are mostly slow-twitch fibers that can work for a long time without tiring. That's essential, because these are the muscles responsible for helping keep you upright. The slow-twitch muscles that make up the bulk of your pelvic floor are that kind of slow-to-tire, persistently supportive muscles.

Fast-twitch fibers, by contrast, provide the quick forcefulness of sprinters. The muscles that move your eyes, for example, are fast-twitch muscles. In the pelvic floor, the fast-twitch muscles assist in controlling the contraction and relaxation that open and close the bladder and bowel and that serve the sexual function so essentially.

While both the slow-twitch and fast-twitch muscles lose strength as the body ages, the fast-twitch muscle fibers do so more readily. The slow-twitch muscles that make the pelvic floor a center of endurance and support tend to keep their power and function longer—unless there is trauma or injury. In a sense, the power to endure remains, while the power to perform some of the pelvic floor's key functions can diminish.

That's natural. As we get older, our powers diminish. That's why it's so important to stay as fit as we can for as long as we can; physical strength and vigor are the best defense against the aging process.

That's certainly true where the pelvic floor muscles are concerned. It's no exaggeration to say that a healthy pelvic core is a major component of a healthy you. For that reason, it's important to pay attention to any pelvic pain or disorder; it could be a signal that something may be wrong. And unfortunately, lots of things can go wrong.

PAIN AT THE CORE

Of course, anytime you have a mechanism as highly complex as the pelvic floor, with all those muscles, nerves, tissues, and ligaments holding all those organs and attached to all that bone, it's prone to things going wrong. Basically, however, there are four root causes of pelvic floor disorders: inflammation, infection, trauma, and a range of what we might term "mechanical" muscular conditions—and any number of contributing factors that set the causes in motion.

Any kind of chronic inflammatory condition in any of the pelvic organs can originate a disorder.

So can any kind of infection: urinary tract infection, yeast infection, bacterial infection, or a major disease that affects the area.

Certainly, an injury from an accident or fall can cause dysfunction. Surgery—a hysterectomy, prostatectomy, or Caesarean section—can leave the muscles weak or injured. And physical or sexual abuse may also produce harmful trauma.

But it's equally possible that an individual's pelvic floor disorder has been caused by simple weakness in the trunk and pelvic stabilizers. Or maybe the person's spine and pelvis are misaligned. The individual may simply have been born with these conditions; it's not uncommon to inherit a weak trunk or a spinal misalignment. Or the conditions could be a result of poor posture, excessive strain from heavy lifting or other physical activities, or working at a repetitive-motion job. It is possible that you are using the pelvic floor muscles incorrectly, resulting in incoordination of the muscles. All can overload and/or shorten the pelvic floor muscles. Such stress weakens the muscles and decreases their range of motion.

Moreover, it doesn't take much to throw a monkey wrench into the works and kick off a disorder in the pelvic floor. Something as common as childbirth can do it. So can wearing clothing that is too tight, sliding too hard into third base at the Fourth of July softball game, using the wrong over-the-counter treatment for a yeast infection, or even playing a wind instrument. Any or all of these triggering factors could lead to a spasm or weakness or impairment of the muscles, producing dysfunctions ranging from debilitating pain to irritable bowel syndrome to skin disorders to erectile dysfunction and/or lowered libido.

And here's the problem: precisely because the pelvic floor muscles are so closely interconnected, any kind of disorder anywhere in the pelvic floor can have an impact on any or all of the pelvic floor's other functions. You might strain a muscle during a gym workout and find that you are having a hard time fighting urinary urgency and a painful time having sex with your partner—all from a spasm suffered during spinning class!

This is the heart of the matter: one pelvic floor dysfunction may lead to another. And another. And still another. One disorder anywhere might therefore cause disabling pain, incontinence, urinary and bowel retention, and sexual dysfunction—often, all at once.

What's more, since the pelvic floor connects our upper and lower body, a dysfunction in the floor can, unfortunately, affect both upper and lower body. I've treated patients for pelvic floor disorder who then reported that their foot pain or back pain disappeared with the treatment. The reason? Pain from their pelvic floor had radiated downward or upward to affect these other areas of the body.

In fact, that's typical. All those muscles, nerves, tissues, and ligaments networked together in support of the pelvic organs simply turn into speedy highways for the pain from a pelvic floor dysfunction. What starts at the core is soon cascading every which way throughout your body. That's why so many people who suffer from a pelvic floor disorder feel a combination of symptoms, and it's why their suffering may not stop at the pelvic region.

And it's the main reason why pelvic floor disorder is rarely the first thing we think of for the range of symptoms the disorder can prompt. A case of diarrhea may send us to the Pepto Bismol bottle or the gastroenterologist. Vaginal pain prompts us to make an appointment with the gynecologist. And back pain is typically a signal to go see an orthopedist or lie down for a couple of days with some heat and ice.

The problem is compounded by the fact that once in the doctor's office, many pelvic floor disorders are often diagnosed as a problem in the organ. They *feel like* organ pain even if there's no infection there, and they can mimic organ disorders, so that's what doctors tend to treat, even though the pain is actually radiating out from a dysfunction in the muscle, tissue, nerve, ligament, or all of them.

Wherever it hurts, these dysfunctions can affect the quality of life in the most intimate arenas of life; at their worst, their impact can make the individual utterly miserable every minute of the day.

CONSEQUENCES OF PELVIC FLOOR DISORDERS

Think what can happen if the pelvic floor no longer performs its vital functions well. If the organs of the pelvis—reproductive organs, bladder, bowel—are not well supported against gravity and cushioned against pressure, they literally may begin to drop. As they sag, they fail to work properly, and pressure and pain may ensue. Incontinence may result. And finally, surgery may be required.

If the muscles that control the urges and openings for evacuation grow weak or are impaired, the result will be difficulty in either evacuating or retaining—or both. You'll experience strain, bloating, diarrhea, and abdominal and/or pelvic pain. You may suffer incontinence and a range of other urinary and bowel symptoms as well.

If the muscles that power sexual activity grow weak or are over-tensed, your ability to respond to your partner will be diminished—and so will your enjoyment and your partner's. At worst, if the tension is really bad, penetration may prove painful, even impossible, for the woman, while men may suffer pain following ejaculation.

ENDING THE PAIN, HEALING THE DISORDER

The whole subject of pelvic pain may be one you're uncomfortable talking about—to your partner, a friend, even to your doctor. Maybe you assumed that the pain or discomfort would subside, then go away in time. Or maybe you've decided it's just something you have to learn to live with.

No, you don't. In fact, you shouldn't.

My program of natural healing is about solutions to your pain that you can do yourself. When I work with patients one-on-one in my physical therapy studio, I prescribe strengthening, stretching, and relaxation exercises, modifications to diet and lifestyle behavior, and the application of manual techniques, biofeedback, deep massage, heat and cold, and the other specialized treatment methods of physical therapy. I've adapted all those modalities, as we call them in physical therapy, into a program you can do at home, by yourself, without having to take medication or buy special equipment.

The exercise program consists of a set of simple movements you can do both in the privacy of your house and throughout the day, wherever you are; you'll learn them in a phased approach. You'll also find nutritional recommendations aimed at alleviating your discomfort and suggestions for home spa treatments that let you soothe your discomfort and pamper yourself.

And the fact is that what you learn in this book can do more than end your pain and cure your disorder. These exercises and self-care therapies can also help you forestall the effects of aging. They can help you enhance the physical intimacy you enjoy with your partner. They can give you a new level of physical strength at the core that will translate into a better sense of well-being in every aspect of your life.

Are you ready to begin?

CHAPTER 2

WHEN THE PELVIC FLOOR IS NOT HEALTHY

Maybe you sat too long on that concrete stadium bench during the rock concert. The result is a pain in the tailbone that just won't go away. After a time, you're feeling it in your lower back as well. It seems to throw your body off balance so that when you stand up, you favor your right side, and when you walk, you more or less have to hunch over. All of that seems to have sent the discomfort into your hip and upper leg.

What's more, you notice that you're racing to the bathroom more frequently than ever, propelled by a feeling of real urgency. If you cough or even laugh, you actually leak, and you wonder if you're growing incontinent.

You would complain to your spouse, but the two of you seem to be growing apart as your sex life has gone south. The reason? You're just feeling too much pain to engage in sex, much less enjoy it.

If this sounds like a far-fetched description of what can happen if you sit on a hard surface for too long, it isn't. The fact is that prolonged sitting is one of the many seemingly ordinary activities that can cause pelvic floor dysfunction.

Of course, it's also possible to have just one distressing symptom. An avid runner with a weak pelvic floor may find herself leaking every time she goes for a run or coughs or sneezes or picks up her baby. But the distinctive character of pelvic floor dysfunction is that pain that starts in one small area from one single cause can spread throughout the muscles, tissues, nerves, and organs of your pelvis, up and down your body, and into your central nervous system, causing more irritation that causes further pain—and possibly confusing your doctor.

THE VICIOUS CIRCLE OF PELVIC PAIN

So any kind of disorder anywhere in the pelvic floor can have an impact on any or all of the pelvic floor's other functions. Once a cascade of deterioration is set in motion, each new difficulty makes it harder to cure the original disorder and/or alleviate the pain.

To get a more in-depth understanding of this cascade, let's start by dividing pelvic floor disorders into two major categories—musculoskeletal pain disorders and bladder, bowel, and sexual dysfunctions. The problem is that a dysfunction or an irritation or pain in one of the two types can cause a dysfunction or an irritation and pain in the other type. That is, a disorder in the muscles or skeleton can cause a bladder, bowel, and/or sexual disorder—and vice versa.

So a bladder infection might end up causing you terrible pain in your legs, while a strained groin muscle could lead to uncomfortable bowel retention and bloating. Bruise your tailbone at the stadium concert—a musculoskeletal disorder—and you may eventually experience bladder and bowel disorders plus sexual dysfunction. By the same token, something as simple as a case of constipation or diarrhea can cause spasm, tightening, or shortening of the musculoskeletal tissue in the pelvic floor, and that in turn can cause pain up and down your core, back, legs, genital area, groin, and hips.

What's particularly vicious about this is that as the infection or inflammation or injury gets worse, it may cause the muscles to tighten and shorten. And as that happens, the pelvic floor musculature gets overloaded and grows weak. With the capabilities of the pelvic floor thus limited, the symptoms of the original infection or inflammation or injury become even worse. As if that weren't enough, the infection and inflammation may also cause scarring in the tissue. The scar tissue can adhere around muscles, nerves, or organs, which may further decrease your mobility and lead to even greater pain. It's really a no-win situation.

So let's look at the different kinds of dysfunctions, irritations, and pain in each of the two main components of pelvic disorder—musculoskeletal disorder and bladder/bowel/sexual disorders—one at a time. (For detailed information on all the dysfunctions and disorders of the pelvic floor, see Appendix A at the end of the book.)

Musculoskeletal Aches and Pains

Musculoskeletal disorders range from bones being out of alignment to muscles feeling knotted, tight, tired, or weak to nerve irritation. The pain can be local, or it can radiate to other parts of the body. For example, pain from an irritated nerve might be felt all along the nerve. Misalignment of the back or pelvis can aggravate nerves which then aggravate the surrounding muscles and tissues. It may hurt to exert yourself—either in one spot or all over, or you just might feel you don't have the strength to do so. You might be sensitive to even slight pressure applied near the ache; it may feel tender or painful. Or maybe you feel the pain as a spasm when you move or as a dull, persistent nuisance.

The pain might be in your lower back, thighs, abdomen, pubic area, genital region, groin, hips, butt, sit bone, or right in the pelvis. Tailbone pain is common; radiating to your gluteal muscles, it can make it difficult to sit. Or perhaps the pain has started in the tailbone but has spread throughout the muscles at the bottom of the pelvic floor to the rectum. That makes it difficult or painful to urinate or defecate.

A dull ache when you're standing up for a while may mean that the blood veins in your pelvic area are congested—that is, the blood has accumulated in the veins and doesn't flow well. In addition to the pain, you may feel either an urgency to urinate or difficulty emptying the bladder or bowel. Women may find it too painful to have sexual intercourse, while men may experience erectile dysfunction or postcoital pain.

Women can have some pelvic floor disorders that are particular to them. In addition to painful intercourse, women can suffer pelvic cavity infections and inflammations that scar and adversely affect their reproductive organs. Endometriosis is one of the most common of these pelvic inflammatory diseases. In addition, women also suffer some very particular vulvar discomforts, including the burning and irritation known as vulvodynia and vaginismus, the inability to undergo vaginal penetration—during sex, with a tampon, or during a medical examination. With vulvar vestibulitis, the skin on the outside portal of the vagina becomes red and highly irritated; the slightest touch can cause severe pain.

In addition, menstrual pain, with its distinctive cramping, tends to tense a woman's muscles, and that in turn can significantly restrict the muscles of the abdomen and pelvic floor.

Women also suffer a range of skin conditions that can result in or be a result of tightening or shortening of the pelvic floor muscles. Skin inflammations or eruptions that cause lesions and adhesions may scar and narrow the vagina, making intercourse even more painful.

There are also musculoskeletal pelvic floor disorders particular to men. In fact, the most common prostate problems, prostatitis and prostadynia, can result in, contribute to, or be caused by pelvic floor disorders—and can be alleviated using the natural healing methods described in this book.

Bladder and Bowel Disorders

Bladder and bowel discomfort seems to come in two different forms. There's the discomfort of fullness and the discomfort of excessive emptying out. With the former, you feel bloated. You might have gas or constipation. It's hard to begin to void. You may feel pressure and pain, and you have the sense that you cannot empty yourself—or it hurts when you try.

With the latter, it's almost the exact opposite. This time, the pressure is an urgency to go, and you find you're going often. You might have diarrhea, or maybe you're getting out of bed multiple times during the night to race to the toilet.

Bladder Disorders. Bladder disorders—for example, interstitial cystitis—are common to both men and women, and in both, they can cause urinary frequency, urgency, retention, and recurring pain that may affect the genital area, the back, and the abdomen. Incontinence may eventually result from these bladder disorders.

What's going on?

What happens is that irritation in the lining of the bladder or in the muscle or nerve irritates the surrounding tissues as well, including the musculoskeletal tissue. That's the vicious circle at work again. If the irritation persists, the muscle tightens and shortens, and that in turn causes more irritation and more pain.

Typically, the person will try to relieve the irritation by urinating. If this happens enough, the brain learns to accompany the irritation with the need to urinate. Eventually, the person gets tired of the frequent trips to the bathroom and will try to hold it in. That tightens the pelvic floor muscles, and those muscles shorten and tighten even more. And that, in turn, acts like a belt tightening around the bladder, giving the person the feeling of needing to urinate even when the bladder is not full. So the vicious circle is simply exacerbated.

Bowel Disorders. Common symptoms of abnormal bowel function in both men and women sound a lot like bladder discomfort: frequency, urgency, retention, spasms, pressure, difficulty with initiation, incontinence. But to these we must add gas, constipation, diarrhea, inflammatory bowel, and irritable bowel syndrome. The effect of these disorders ranges from the extremely unpleasant to the intensely painful. Inflammations of the bowel can affect all layers of the intestine and rectum, while the group of symptoms involved in irritable bowel syndrome can cause considerable abdominal pain.

What's more, most of these disorders can produce increased toxins in the gut, which in turn irritates the surrounding tissues, including the musculoskeletal tissue. As with bladder irritations, persistent irritation may tighten and shorten the muscles, which will create more irritation and more pain—not just in the pelvis but through the abdomen, back, legs, and buttocks.

Of course, any of these disorders can limit your daily activity. And the worse the resulting pain, the less active and social you become, and the more homebound and inactive your life.

THE IMPACT: WHAT PELVIC FLOOR DISORDERS CAN DO TO YOU

Pelvic floor disorders can be painful, disruptive, and emotionally stressful and upsetting. If misdiagnosed, as they frequently are, they may lead to unnecessary and therefore destructive drug therapies or even surgical procedures. Even without such extreme effects, these disorders can cause life-changing results—including organ prolapse, incontinence, skin disorders, and sexual dysfunction.

Prolapsed Organs

Organ prolapse takes place when the pelvic floor musculature and tissues become so strained from irritation, infection, inflammation, weakness, or trauma that the organs of the pelvis literally fall. In both men and women, the rectum may fall into the back wall of the pelvis. In women, the bladder may collapse downward and backward into the front wall of the vagina. The uterus can descend, and it can take the vaginal vault with it. The urethra may collapse as well. The pouchlike space between the rectum and the back wall of the uterus might be displaced, potentially causing pressure, pain, or the feeling that something is actually falling out of you.

Often with prolapsed organs, the pain is not immediate and not severe or nonexistent, so people may have no idea they have the condition.

Incontinence

Incontinence of both bladder and bowel can be a common result of pelvic floor disorder, mostly resulting from weakness or shortening of the muscle. It comes in several forms.

In urinary stress incontinence, a cough or sneeze, lifting, or running can cause sudden involuntary urine loss. As many as 38 percent of women engaging in high-impact athletics experience stress incontinence during the athletic activity.

Different from stress incontinence, urge incontinence is characterized by a quick warning that precedes the strong desire to void that results in the involuntary urine loss. A great many women and men also suffer from a combination of both stress and urge incontinence. And many also experience fecal incontinence, typically due to weak or shortened muscles in the pelvic floor.

Skin Conditions

A cascade of skin conditions, such as lichen sclerosus and lichen planus, can result in pelvic floor disorder, and pelvic floor disorder may contribute to the discomfort of such skin conditions. It's another case of the revolving door effect—the vicious circle of pelvic floor disorder. These skin conditions may derive from a compromised immune system, from sexually transmitted diseases, and sometimes from the inappropriate use of vaginal creams. Or, the condition may be congenital—that is, you're just born with it.

Whether a contributing cause of pelvic floor disorder or a result of it, these conditions can be unpleasant, painful, and disfiguring.

Sexual Dysfunction

Pelvic floor disorders cause a range of sexual dysfunctions. To begin with, these disorders can greatly decrease libido in both men and women. If arousal does happen, both men and women may find it difficult or even impossible to achieve orgasm due to weak or overly shortened muscles.

In a condition known as dyspareunia, women may feel pain during intercourse. This pain is in the initial penetration, or with deep penetration, or from the thrusting motion, or from a lack of lubrication. Superficial scarring, adhesions, skin irritation, or muscle tenderness may all contribute to the pain and discomfort.

In men, erectile dysfunction can be a direct result of pelvic floor muscle tension, weakness, or pelvic congestion. Or it may result from experiencing pain during or after intercourse.

HEALING YOUR PELVIC FLOOR DISORDER

It is essential to get a proper diagnosis from a specialist in pelvic floor dysfunction, because, as you can see, the list of things that can go wrong with your pelvic floor is a long one, covering a varied range of complex signs, symptoms, and dysfunctions. I've included such a list as Appendix A to this book. Consult it about any sign or symptom that you think may be related to or radiating from the core of your body—and take action accordingly.

Whatever kind of pelvic pain you're suffering, and whatever the particular pelvic floor disorder that afflicts you, I'm certain you're eager to start the natural healing that can ease the pain and alleviate the disorder.

There are two separate exercise programs, depending on whether your problem is pain—and the accompanying bladder or bowel discomfort—or weakness. Each of these programs consists of different exercise routines, and each progresses in phases.

The first program is the End-the-Pain routine, a three-phased course that focuses on what I'm sure is most important to you right now—your pain. The entire End-the-Pain routine must also be accompanied by the external and internal massages described in Chapter 5. Do these two therapies together to ensure an end to your pain.

The second exercise program addresses the problem of weakness—specifically, bladder and bowel incontinence and decreased sexual pleasure. The Strengthen-the-Muscles routine is in four phases.

For both exercise programs, you'll progress from one phase to the next only after you've become comfortable with the earlier phase and have begun to feel its benefits. The Symptoms Monitor at the end of this chapter is your tool for assessing when it's time to move on.

If you have symptoms of both pain and weakness, begin your healing with the End-the-Pain routine and the massage therapies of Chapter 5, and move on to the exercises of the Strengthen-the-Muscles routine only when you are 100 percent pain-free—and assuming you still have an incontinence problem. It is very often the case that the exercises of the End-the-Pain routine will end your incontinence as well, so you may not feel the need to do the other strengthening routine. Or, you may decide to do just some of those exercises in order to keep your muscles strong and stave off a return of incontinence.

If you succeed in healing your pain through the End-the-Pain routine and the self-massage you'll learn in Chapter 5, then begin the Strengthen-the-Muscles routine only to find that some pain symptoms have again surfaced, stop! Go back to the End-the-Pain routine. In other words, it's important to be pain-free when you undertake the strengthening exercises to address problems of incontinence.

Be sure also that you take note of any negative responses as you change exercises or increase the intensity of any exercise—for example, by doing more repetitions or by adding resistance—or as you move from phase to phase in a routine. By negative responses, I mean an increase in the level of pain or a worsening of the disorder's symptoms. If such responses do occur, first check your posture and alignment; that is, make sure you're doing the exercise correctly. Then, cut back on the intensity of the exercise: do fewer repetitions or use less resistance. If you still feel the negative response, go back to the earlier part of the End-the-Pain routine. If none of this helps, you should by all means contact your health-care provider.

Chances are you won't have any negative responses. If you follow the phased programs carefully, your healing will progress. The pain will diminish and then end, and your weakness will turn to strength.

I'm sure you're eager to get started. Task number one is to fill out the following Symptoms Monitor. It's a questionnaire that asks you to pinpoint where it hurts, how much it hurts, and what effect the pain or incontinence and other symptoms are having on your life. You'll use this Symptoms Monitor over the next weeks and months as a guide to advance from phase to phase in each program. With today's assessment, you'll create a baseline. Come back to the Symptoms Monitor four weeks from now to reassess your symptoms. If your symptoms have improved by 50 percent or more, you are ready to move to the next phase of the program. If your improvement is less than 50 percent, wait another four weeks, then try again. Keep reassessing your pain and symptoms every four weeks as you do the natural healing exercises and other therapies of this book; you'll see as well as feel the improvement.

SYMPTOMS MONITOR

The following questionnaire is reproduced with permission from the International Pelvic Pain Society, www.pelvicpain.org.

For each question, circle 0, 1, 2, 3, 4, or 5 where, for pain, 0 = no pain and 5 = severe pain, and for non-pain symptoms, 0 = no symptoms and 5 = severe symptoms.

Pain

How would you rate your present pain?	0	1	2	3	4	5
Pain when lifting?	0	1	2	3	4	5
Pain when sitting?	0	1	2	3	4	5
Pain when walking?	0	1	2	3	4	5
Pain while doing physical activity?	0	1	2	3	4	5
Deep pain with intercourse or sexual activity?	0	1	2	3	4	5
Pelvic pain lasting hours or days after sexual activity?	0	1	2	3	4	5
Pain when bladder is full?	0	1	2	3	4	5
Pain with urination?	0	1	2	3	4	5
Pain after urination?	0	1	2	3	4	5
Muscle or joint pain?	0	1	2	3	4	5
Abdominal pain?	0	1	2	3	4	5
Backache?	0	1	2	3	4	5
Pain when wearing tight clothing?	0	1	2	3	4	5
Pain with bowel movement?	0	1	2	3	4	5

Pain after bowel movement?	0	1	2	3	4	5
A falling-out feeling or a feeling of pressure in the pelvis?	0	1	2	3	4	5

For Women Only

Pain at ovulation (midcycle) ?	0	1	2	3	4	5
Pain level just before period?	0	1	2	3	4	5
Pain (not cramps) with period?	0	1	2	3	4	5
Cramps with period?	0	1	2	3	4	5
Pain after period is over?	0	1	2	3	4	5
Burning vaginal pain with penetration of tampon or during sex?	0	1	2	3	4	5
Difficulty achieving orgasm (even when aroused)?	0	1	2	3	4	5

For Men Only

Difficulty getting an erection (even when aroused)?	0	1	2	3	4	5
Difficulty achieving orgasm (even when aroused)?	0	1	2	3	4	5

Bladder Symptoms

Loss of urine when coughing, sneezing, lifting, or laughing?	0	1	2	3	4	5
Frequency of urination versus the norm of once every two to three hours?	0	1	2	3	4	5

Urgency or need to urinate with little warning?	0	1	2	3	4	5
Loss of urine due to strong urge?	0	1	2	3	4	5
Difficulty initiating urine stream?	0	1	2	3	4	5
Urine stream stops and starts?	0	1	2	3	4	5
Nighttime urinary frequency?	0	1	2	3	4	5
Incomplete emptying of urine?	0	1	2	3	4	5

Bowel Symptoms

Constipation (fewer than three bowel movements a week)?	0	1	2	3	4	5
Bowel frequency (more than three bowel movements a day)?	0	1	2	3	4	5
Incomplete emptying of bowel?	0	1	2	3	4	5
Urgency or need to have a bowel movement with little warning?	0	1	2	3	4	5
Abdominal bloating or fullness?	0	1	2	3	4	5
Lumpy or hard stool consistency?	0	1	2	3	4	5
Loose or watery stool consistency?	0	1	2	3	4	5
Needing to strain to achieve bowel movement?	0	1	2	3	4	5
Fecal incontinence?	0	1	2	3	4	5

Effect on Daily Life

Since your symptoms began, how much has your lifestyle been affected? (0 = not at all and 5 = substantive change)

Symptoms or pain limit or interfere with work or school?	0	1	2	3	4	5
Symptoms or pain limit or interfere with social activities?	0	1	2	3	4	5
Symptoms or pain limit or interfere with exercise routine?	0	1	2	3	4	5
Symptoms or pain limit such activities as lifting, cleaning, carrying things, shopping, etc.?	0	1	2	3	4	5
Symptoms or pain limit or interfere with recreational and/or athletic activities?	0	1	2	3	4	5
Symptoms or pain limit or interfere with sexual activity?	0	1	2	3	4	5
Symptoms or pain disrupt sleep?	0	1	2	3	4	5
Symptoms or pain cause unexplained mood changes?	0	1	2	3	4	5

Baseline assessment point total: _____

Start date: _____

Reassessment Date   **Point Total**

_____   _____

_____   _____

_____   _____

_____   _____

_____   _____

_____   _____

CHAPTER 3

END THE PAIN

Do this program of exercises to treat any musculoskeletal pain in the abdomen, back, thigh, hip, genital, or pelvic region and/or any pain or abnormal symptoms associated with urination or defecation, or with sexual activity. This may include the following:

In Both Men and Women
- Tailbone pain: spasm or tension in butt or pelvic floor muscles
- Pudendal neuralgia: irritation or pain that typically worsens with sitting and is felt along the nerve pathways from the lower back to the rectal area, the genital area, and/or the bladder
- Pain in the lower back, sacroiliac joint, hip, groin, and/or pelvis
- Interstitial cystitis/painful bladder syndrome
- Irritable bowel syndrome and/or colitis (including constipation and diarrhea)
- Urge urinary or bowel incontinence (strong, sudden need to evacuate with leakage)
- Urinary or bowel urgency, frequency (including nighttime frequency, or nocturia), retention, or difficulty with initiation

- Feeling of fullness, abdominal pressure and/or pain
- Urethral or rectal spasms, burning, pain, or itching
- Pelvic pain from muscle spasm, nerve irritation, or adhesions
- Decreased libido due to pain and/or contracted or tight pelvic floor muscles
- Difficulty achieving orgasm due to pain and/or contracted or tight pelvic floor muscles
- Genital hyperarousal
- Any other disorder listed in Appendix A that causes any of the symptoms listed here

In Women Only
- Vaginal pain
- Vulvar vestibulitis: irritation and/or inflammation of vestibule to the vagina
- Vaginismus: muscle tension preventing penetration of the vagina
- Dyspareunia: pain during intercourse, superficial or deep, or postcoital pain
- Prenatal or postpartum pelvic pain
- Endometriosis or other pelvic infection or inflammation
- Dysmenorrhea (painful menstrual periods)
- Difficulty with conception: infertility due to pelvic congestion or scarring

In Men Only
- Erectile dysfunction or postcoital pain
- Prostatodynia or nonbacterial prostatitis (pain in or around the prostate)

The main key to healing your pelvic floor disorder the natural way is to end the pain or discomfort. The program for doing so is in three parts and must be accompanied by the massage therapies described in Chapter 5.

In Part 1 of the End-the-Pain routine, you'll learn to let go—to relax your muscles, relieve them of any tension and strain, let them pause and come to rest. A routine of 11 simple exercises will help you do all that—the essential first step toward healing the disorder at your core.

In Part 2, you'll concentrate on strengthening your core with four other exercises added to the routine.

In both Parts 1 and 2, you'll also undertake some basic cardiovascular activity as a way of maintaining overall fitness and keeping your immune system strong.

Then in Part 3, you'll begin integrating some of your normal recreational or athletic activities back into your life, monitoring how it feels and what impact, if any, it has on your pain or symptoms.

How long will each part last? That depends entirely on you—on how bad your pain and other symptoms are, on their underlying cause, on your general level of health and fitness, and of course on how you respond to the program of exercises. Keep in mind that you are an absolutely unique individual in every way, including in what works for you in terms of your body.

In general, however, it might take anywhere from one month to as many as four months for the Letting Go exercises of Part 1 to make a difference. That sounds like a long time, but the truth is that it isn't easy to learn to relax the muscles, especially muscles that you may have automatically been clenching for some time. In other words, it took a long while to tighten and shorten those muscles, and it's going to take some time to loosen and lengthen them as well.

Still, once you do achieve the letting go and begin to feel relief from your symptoms, things move more swiftly. You'll start seeing the benefits of the strengthening exercises of Part 2 in one or two months. *Do not do the advanced exercises in Part 2 until you are free from pain and need a challenge.*

And so long as you ease back into your recreational activity and keep a close watch on your progress, you may feel the rewards of Part 3 in a matter of weeks. If, however, your symptoms do not improve or if they improve but are still present after six months of this routine, see a specialist in pelvic floor dysfunction.

I know you're eager to begin, so let's start letting go.

PART I: LETTING GO

You have to work at relaxing. That sounds ironic, of course, but it's true.

The reason is that tensing our muscles may be an automatic reaction. We do it so often, so spontaneously, for so long that the tension settles into our bodies and the tightness becomes the norm. We don't even know we're tense.

Ever have one of those days when you didn't even realize how keyed up you were till your friend or spouse or maybe a considerate coworker started kneading your neck and shoulder muscles? Wow! You could almost feel the tension flowing out of you, and it felt delicious.

The truth is you tend to tense your muscles throughout the course of the day. We all do. It's a subconscious response to the various stresses, strains, and annoyances we encounter—to the sheer tumult of daily life. Maybe you tense your shoulders and end up with a stiff neck and clenched jaw. Maybe you feel the stress in your lower back. Or maybe, like so many of us, the tension tends to settle in the bottom of your core, right in the muscles of the pelvic floor. The tensing shortens the muscles, and that weakens them. Result? That vicious circle of pelvic floor pain and dysfunction is set in motion.

The key to healing, therefore, is to let go of the tension so we can stretch and elongate the pelvic floor muscles, then strengthen the muscles around them. This strengthening of the surrounding muscles provides support to the pelvic floor muscles so they don't have to work so hard. That's why most of the Letting Go exercises are about stretching, and it's why most of the stretches focus on the external muscles of the hip, back, pelvic, and abdominal areas. The reason?

Tightness and weakness in these muscles can make it difficult to do the simplest activities—walking, for instance—and that, in turn, can throw you off balance. Being off balance, of course, just tightens and weakens the muscles further, and pretty soon, you're caught in the vicious circle of pelvic floor pain and disorder.

Stretching increases the flexibility of the tissues being stretched. It helps to loosen the tension in your muscles, de-stresses them, and thus helps you manage your mental stress as well. But there is a right way to stretch and a wrong way, and it's essential to do the stretches of the Letting Go exercises the right way.

The right way is the simple way. The key is to *stretch in a relaxed manner—as you breathe*. You want to be relaxed because over-stretching or stretching too hard may actually injure the muscles further and can even irritate the nerves, causing even more pain. This is especially true if your muscles are knotted to begin with; in that case, your best bet is to massage away the knots first—see Chapter 5. In all cases, you want to breathe as you stretch in order to increase the blood flow and the supply of oxygen to the tissues of the muscles you're stretching.

As you continue to do these stretches, you will begin to notice that you are able to stretch farther. It means your muscles are loosening and lengthening. It means the exercises are working and the healing is beginning.

Getting Started on Letting Go Exercises

Done in sequence in a relaxed manner, the Letting Go exercises take less than half an hour. Do the exercises in conjunction with the sore points self-massage you'll learn in Chapter 5; this will only add a few minutes to your total time. Start every day with this routine, making it as automatic a part of your morning as brushing your teeth.

In addition, repeat the exercises at intervals during the day. Two of the first four—deep breathing and the pelvic drop—can be done pretty much anywhere without drawing undue attention to yourself. The pelvic floor stretch, the thigh press, and Steps 5 through 11, however, will require a quiet, preferably private environment.

Again, don't go at these exercises like a hard-charging fullback in a football game. Don't do more than is asked; stick to the recommended number of seconds to hold a stretch and don't do more than the recommended number of repetitions. If you are in severe pain, you may even be well advised to start with fewer repetitions and to hold each for fewer seconds than recommended. Sometimes, less really is better. Be good to your body; it deserves it.

In addition to doing the 11 exercises daily, it's important for you to undertake some form of cardiovascular exercise every day. Cardiovascular exercise is any exercise that increases the flow of blood the heart is pumping—essential to making the healing process as effective as possible. The exercise you choose is up to you. Maybe you're a Rollerblader, or like to work out on the elliptical machine at the gym, or enjoy taking a bike ride. All are great exercises, although if you find it painful to sit, the bike ride may not work out.

Perhaps the simplest as well as one of the best cardiovascular exercises is walking. I don't mean strolling, and I don't mean the walking you do as you struggle home from the store with your arms loaded with packages. I mean walking that you set out to do as an exercise—at a steady pace that is fast but comfortable, for at least five and up to 60 continuous minutes. Five minutes is a good start if you have not been doing any exercise lately, but if you're a fairly active person, half an hour is a good beginning, and you can work your way up from there. If you can't do 30 minutes all at once, by all means do less, but walk twice a day so that you build up your endurance. In due course, you'll be taking a 30-minute walk and feeling fine about it.

In addition to the walking or any other cardio exercise routine, keep the heart pumping and the blood flowing by regularly standing up from your desk or turning off the laptop or putting the baby down for a nap and walking around for a few minutes—purposefully and at a good pace. Do this at least three times a day—five times is better—to get the blood flowing back into the legs, buttocks, and pelvis. And as you do your cardio or any other form of exercise, remember to breathe. Learning how is the first step toward letting go, ending your pain, and healing your pelvic floor disorder.

Step 1: Breathe

Not just breathe: deep-breathe. That is a very different thing from the unthinking taking in and letting out of air that every living being does willy-nilly. Very often, such spontaneous breathing is just shallow breathing: typically only the upper part of the lungs is being put to work, and not enough oxygen gets into the system.

Even some so-called deep breathing can be shallow. When the doctor tells you to "take a deep breath," do you suck in your stomach and lift up your shoulders? If so, you're breathing shallowly.

To see what I mean, picture the lungs as a two-part bladder with an upper and lower chamber. When you suck in your belly to take that deep breath the doctor ordered, you're actually creating a partial vacuum in the lower chamber of your lungs, sweeping all the air into the upper chamber. That's why you have to raise your shoulders. But all you've really taken in is enough air to fill the upper chamber. Your lungs are half full.

Here's how to do true deep breathing:

1. *Inhale.* Expand your belly outward and your ribs to the sides, and "open" your pelvic floor, without lifting your chest. Feel the air filling the "receiving area" of your lungs, making one big chamber.
2. *Exhale.* Obviously, you'll do the reverse as you exhale. Start from the top. Let the air out of your upper lungs, then relax your ribs, your belly, and your pelvic floor, so that the air just gradually flows out of you.

Try it. The breathing should be slow and deep. Take three to five seconds to perform the inhalation, then pause for one second. Take even longer—four to six seconds—to do the exhalation, and again, pause for one second. Do it five times.

Start every day with five deep-breathing repetitions, and practice it throughout the day every day—during a work break, before you turn the key in the ignition, at the mall. In time, deep breathing will become automatic. But do deep breathing *consciously* to start your day—and certainly as you perform your pelvic floor exercises and stretches.

Step 2: Drop

The drop is really a breathe-and-drop combination, but the key to it is what is called the pelvic floor drop. If the term sounds a little odd, it's actually something you already know how to do. In fact, this step is as much an intellectual or mental exercise as it is physical, for what you do to drop your pelvic floor is to copy in a conscious way a feeling that is universal to us all—namely, the sensation you feel as you urinate and the urine streams out. You know what it's like: you feel the urge to urinate, but there is nowhere to go until you get home or arrive at the office or turn off the interstate to find a gas station with a working lavatory. The feeling I'm talking about is that moment of relief when you have reached the bathroom; you can finally relax the muscles and let go.

That's the feeling you'll consciously copy in doing the pelvic floor drop.

How do you perform this copycat act? The key is visualization, but deep breathing helps it happen. Here's how:

1. Stand, sit, or lie down—whatever works for you; you may need to try varying positions before you find the one that suits you. Relax your body as much as possible. Close your eyes.

2. Do a conscious deep-breathing inhalation—for three, four, five seconds.

3. Start your exhale. As you do, *visualize* your breath descending the chambers of your lungs and being pressed downward and out from your pelvis as you simply drop those pelvic floor muscles and let go. Don't push or strain; just drop. Breathe out for four to six seconds. Do five repetitions, throughout the day.

If this visualization doesn't work right away, here's a tip: the next few times you urinate, try to remember to capture the feeling you feel when the stream begins to flow. That is the feeling you want to recall and reproduce for this exercise.

The pelvic floor drop is an absolute prerequisite of a healthy pelvic floor. Do it every morning, of course, in combination with your deep breathing, but don't stop there. Do the drop any time and at all times throughout the day—at the office, waiting for the train, while window-shopping, when you feel the urge to void. If there's any tension anywhere in your body, this will help release it.

Step 3: Thigh Press

This simple and very gentle isometric exercise works wonders in helping relax the pelvic floor muscles and calm bladder or bowel urgency and frequency. Over time it helps alleviate pain. But you'll need a private, quiet place to do it.

Lie down on your back—preferably on the floor on a blanket or mat or towel; if not, on your bed if the mattress is firm, with your head resting on a thin pillow. Your knees should be bent; your arms should rest along your sides. Lift your lower legs till they are straight out in front of you, parallel to the floor. Now just raise your hands and place your fingertips atop your thighs, slightly to the outside of the thigh. Very gently, press your fingertips into the thighs; at the same time, let your thighs resist the pressure. Hold

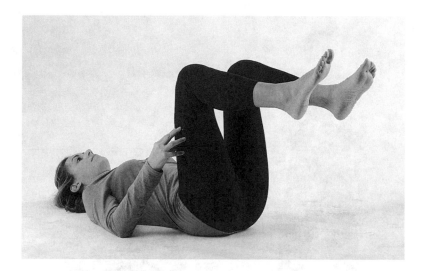

the two-way pressure for five seconds. Relax. Repeat the exercise five times, and do the five reps two to four times a day.

Step 4: Pelvic Floor Stretch

The pelvic floor stretch is a great way to ignite the power of your body's core. It helps open, loosen, and begin to lengthen the pelvic floor—a good foundation for the healing process. There are two ways to do the pelvic floor stretch. If your knees, hips, and back are supple and strong, try it the deep squatting way; if you have trouble squatting or if your butt muscles are knotted, there's an alternate method you can do on your back. Either way you do the pelvic floor stretch, be sure to breathe deeply as you do it.

Here's how to do the squatting stretch:

1. Stand with your legs apart, feet extending a few inches beyond the shoulders, toes turned slightly outward.
2. Keeping your back as straight as possible, squat down till your rear is three to five inches off the floor.

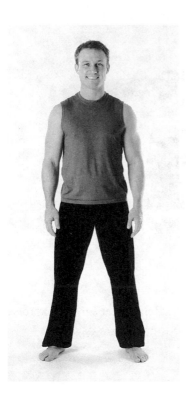
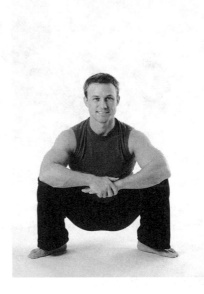

3. Relax into the squat as you do six to eight deep breaths. Your arms should rest inside your thighs, with your hands together or relaxed to the floor.
4. Again keeping your back straight, place your hands on your knees and push yourself up.
5. Hold the stretch for 30 to 60 seconds. Do three repetitions, two to four times a day.

Here's how to do the stretch lying down:

1. Lie on a firm surface—on a mat on the floor or on a hard mattress, as with the thigh press. Bring your knees up to your chest and then let them relax and rotate out to the side so that they flare outward. Use your hands to hold your knees in this position.

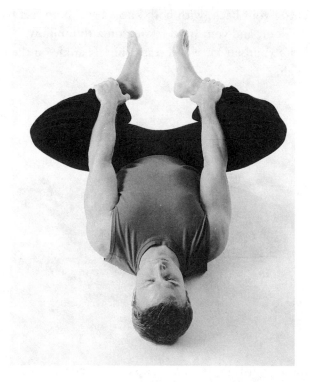

2. Stretch as you deep-breathe for six to eight breaths. Do not bounce, and do not push hard. Just stretch gradually and progressively as you fill and empty your lungs.

3. Hold the stretch for 30 to 60 seconds. Do three repetitions, two to four times a day.

Step 5: Hip Rotator Stretch

Hip rotator muscles do exactly what their name suggests—they enable you to rotate your hip so you can bend and turn. Short, tight hip rotator muscles don't just put stress on your pelvic floor—they also restrict your range of motion. That's why this gentle, steady stretch is so important. Here's how to stretch your hip external rotators:

1. Lie on your back, with both knees bent, both feet flat on the floor, and your head resting on a thin pillow.
2. Raise your left knee and rest your left ankle on the right thigh.

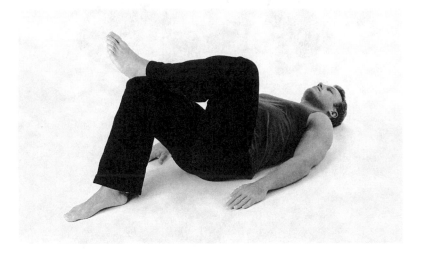

3. Raise your right leg and wrap both hands around the back of your right thigh.
4. Slowly and gently pull your right thigh toward you; you should feel the stretch in the back of your left buttock and

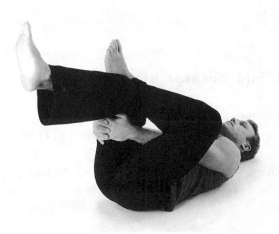

in the hip region. Hold the stretch for a minimum of 30
seconds, maximum of 60 seconds.

5. Repeat with the right leg: right ankle on left thigh, left
leg raised, pull left thigh toward you, hold for 30 to 60
seconds, and feel the stretch in your right buttock and hip
region. Do three repetitions on each side, two to four times
a day.

Step 6: Hip Flexor Stretch

Like the external hip rotators, the hip flexors enable you to raise
your thigh up to your abdomen, to bend, and to flex, as their name
suggests. Here's how to stretch these muscles:

I. Stand straight with feet hip-width apart.

2. Step forward two to three feet with your right foot. The
length of the step forward depends first on how tall you
are—shorter individuals will take a shorter step—and on
how tight your muscles are.

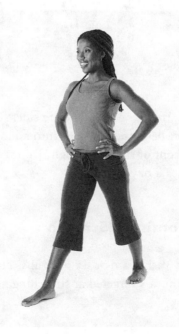

3. Using a chair for balance if you like, and keeping your pelvis square and straight ahead, bend your right knee into a lunge position, making sure that your *right knee does not extend over the toes*; that will strain your knee. You should feel a stretch in the front of the *left* thigh and hip region. If you don't feel a stretch in the front of the left thigh, try extending your right foot farther forward for a deeper lunge, remembering to keep your pelvis square and straight ahead. Hold the stretch for a minimum of 30 and a maximum of 60 seconds.

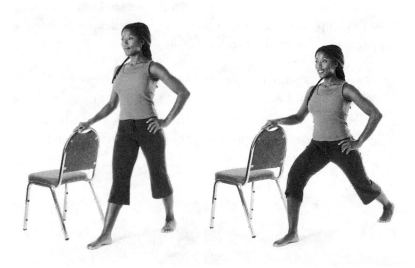

4. Repeat the stretch on the opposite side: step forward with the left foot, bend the left knee into a lunge, feel the stretch along the front of the *right* thigh. Do three repetitions, two to four times a day.

Step 7: Abdominals Stretch

Everybody wants washboard or six-pack abs. The following stretch has a different aim. It's targeted at stretching and lengthening the abdominal muscles that are located just above the pelvic floor and that help support the back. There are two ways to do this stretch—lying flat or standing up. Here's how to do the stretch from a prone position:

1. Lie flat on your stomach on a mat or blanket. Bring your hands up next to your shoulders, palms down.

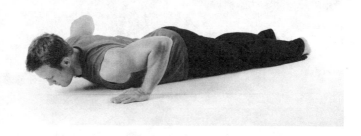

2. Do a deep-breathing inhale.
3. As you exhale, push up slowly on both hands, lifting your upper body, while your hips and legs remain flat. Straighten your arms as much as possible. Hold for 30 to 60 seconds.

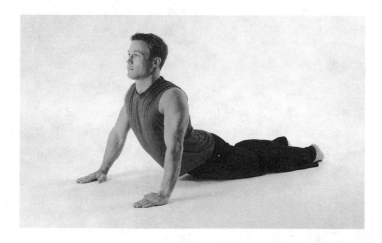

If it's hard for you to straighten your arms, or if you have shoulder, wrist, or elbow problems, try the standing version of the exercise:

1. Stand straight with feet hip-width apart and knees slightly bent. Place your hands on either side of your lower back.

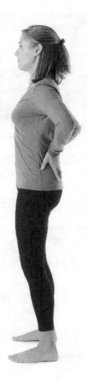

2. Do a deep-breathing inhale.
3. As you exhale, slowly bend your torso backward until you feel a slight stretch in your abs—and possibly in the upper part of your thighs. Hold the stretch for 30 to 60 seconds. Do three repetitions, two to four times a day.

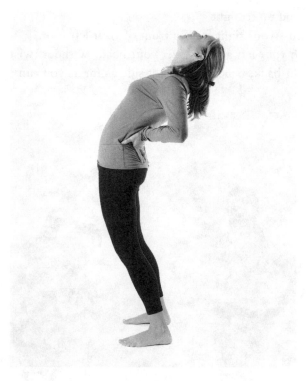

Step 8: Back Stretch

No wonder your back muscles feel tired: you use them nearly all the time. Walking, bending, turning, sitting down, standing up, and of course every sport or physical activity use the back muscles, so these muscles often tighten through sheer fatigue. What's more, the back is a place where tension tends to settle, tightening the muscles even further. There are two ways to stretch, loosen, and lengthen your back muscles, one standing and one lying down. Do whichever one is most comfortable for you, but if you have knee or hip problems, you should not do the lying-down version. Here's the standing version:

1. Stand up straight.
2. Cross your right foot in front of your left foot.
3. Lift your left arm up over your head. Without twisting your back, bend to the right side as far as you can.

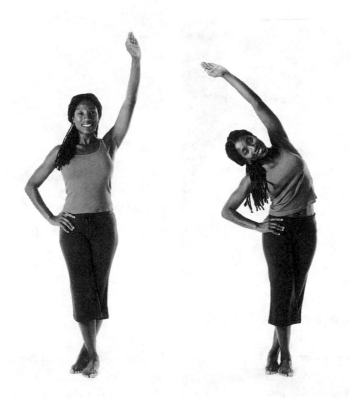

4. Reverse: cross left foot over right foot, raise right arm, bend to the left side. Hold the stretch for 30 to 60 seconds. Do three repetitions on each side, two to four times a day.

And here's the lying-down version:

1. Kneel and then lower your torso so that you are face down with both knees tucked under.

2. Stretch both arms straight out in front of you.

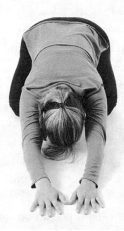

3. Slowly "walk" your hands to the right, curving your torso as you do until you feel a stretch on your left side. Hold the stretch for 30 to 60 seconds.

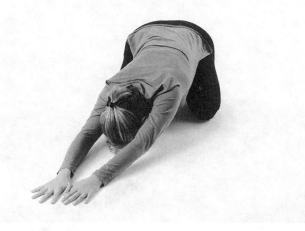

4. Reverse. Walk your hands left till you feel a stretch on your right side.

5. Do three repetitions on each side, two to four times a day.

Step 9: Hamstrings Stretch

The hamstrings are those long muscles behind the knee on the back of the thigh that act on two important joints—your knee and your hip. The hamstrings help those joints extend and flex and are thus crucial in walking, running, jumping, even controlling your torso. So it's important to keep them loose. Here's how:

1. Lie flat on your back with legs straight out in front of you.
2. Raise your left leg straight up and grasp the back of the left thigh with both hands. (Alternatively, wrap a towel around the bottom of your left foot and hold the ends with both hands.)
3. Slowly pull your left leg toward you until you feel a light stretch behind the left thigh. If the stretch hurts, bend the left knee slightly. Hold the stretch for 30 to 60 seconds.

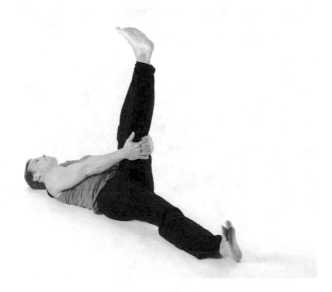

4. Reverse. Raise the right leg and pull it toward you till you feel the stretch behind the right thigh. Do three repetitions on each side, two to four times a day.

Step 10: Inner Thighs Stretch

The muscles of the inner thigh are called adductors, meaning they draw the legs in toward the center of the body. These muscles start at the pelvic bone and attach down the thigh, which is why they provide so much power and stability to the hip area—and why it's so important to keep them flexible. Here's how:

1. Sit on the floor. It might help to sit where your back can line up against a wall behind you, but this is not necessary.
2. With your back straight, draw the balls of your feet together, bending your knees and flaring them outward.

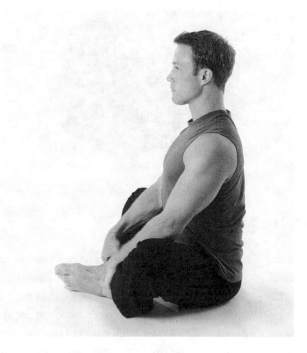

3. Keeping your back straight, slowly lean forward at the hips and press your knees gently toward the floor. Do not overstretch; in time, as you continue to do this stretch, your muscles will lengthen and you will be able to press your

knees closer and closer to the floor (only gymnasts, dancers, or extremely mobile people can get their knees all the way to the floor). Do the usual three reps, holding the stretch for 30 to 60 seconds. Repeat two to four times a day.

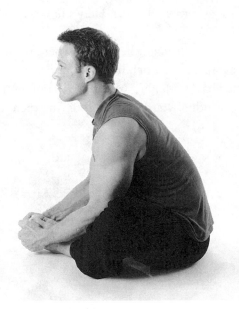

Step II: Butt Stretch

In a society where most of us spend most of our time sitting down, the gluteal muscles—the muscles of the buttocks—tend to grow weak. That's bad, for these are power muscles that help us extend and rotate the hip and torso. Moreover, tension in the gluteal muscles may spread to the lower back and pelvic floor, weakening those muscles, throwing our posture off-kilter, and causing pain. So here's how to loosen and lengthen the gluteal muscles:

1. Lie flat on your back with both legs straight.
2. Bend your right knee up to your chest.

3. With both hands, gently pull the leg closer against your chest. Hold for 30 to 60 seconds.

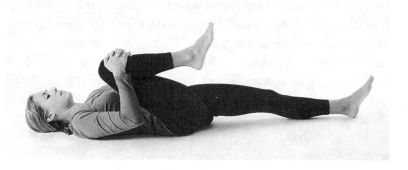

4. Reverse. Bend your left knee and pull it closer against your chest. Do three repetitions on each side, two to four times a day.

Regular Daily Cardio

Don't forget to accompany these exercises with some cardiovascular activity at least once a day. Such exercise—walking, running, biking, climbing, skiing, swimming, aerobics, treadmill workouts, spinning class, and the like—increases the body's blood flow, and that's what helps to keep the organs, tissues, and muscles everywhere in the body healthy.

Cardio exercise also reduces stress and diminishes tension, which can also ease your pain. How? It's called a "natural high." The exercises gets your blood flowing well, and a good flow of blood to the brain increases your production of endorphins, the so-called "natural pain killers" that provide a sense of well-being.

Cardiovascular exercise has many other benefits as well, of course, and these are well known. It can speed up your metabolism, which helps prevent or relieve constipation. It certainly helps control weight, which makes you healthier both physically and emotionally.

It can also be fun.

The important thing about doing cardio during the Letting Go routine in Part 1 is that it be purposeful, sustained, and done regularly. By purposeful, I mean that your walk or bike ride or aerobics routine shouldn't be part of anything else; carve out a special time and devote the time to the exercise. Set a good pace and keep at it steadily. And make sure you do the exercise for at least 5 and up to 60 continuous minutes at least once a day; that is, if you could only exercise for five minutes try to do your five-minute exercise three times a day—for example, before each meal.

As it gets easier, slowly increase your cardio time, although not beyond 60 minutes. Also, if it hurts, stop.

Making the Letting Go Exercises a Part of Your Life

The 11-step Letting Go exercises should be an integral part of your day. In fact, over time, you should try to extend the Letting Go exercises—that is, make your stretches even longer and increase the amount of time you spend doing cardio and the pace of your cardio exercise. Work up to an hour of brisk, sustained cardiovascular activity at least three times a week, preferably five times a week.

Here are my suggestions for making these exercises an integral part of your life:

- Start the day with your half-hour of Letting Go exercises, then take a brisk walk or do a cardio workout—for at least five minutes, preferably 30 or more—before breakfast.
- Do Steps 1 and 2—breathe and drop—throughout the day whenever and wherever you can.
- Then do the 11-exercise routine again, if possible, before lunch, before dinner, and before bed.
- End your prelunch and predinner exercise routines with a brisk walk or other cardio exercise.

- Stick to this schedule, and I'm sure that you'll soon begin to notice your muscles loosening and lengthening and your overall fitness and sense of well-being increasing. Above all, you'll feel relief from your pain—more and more relief each day and week that you do the routine. It means the healing has begun.
- Give it some time to work. Keep track of your progress by filling out the Symptoms Monitor at the end of Chapter 2 once every four weeks. Set a date and time for this: every first Tuesday morning or Saturday afternoon of the month, for example. Only by "keeping score" regularly can you really gauge your progress. Once your pain has gone down by at least 50 percent and your symptoms have improved, you're ready for Part 2 of the End-the-Pain routine.

Part I Schedule

Letting Go exercises: on awakening, before lunch, before dinner, before bed

Cardio: aim for 60 minutes a day, start with at least five.

Breathe and drop exercises: repeatedly throughout the day

PART 2: STRENGTHENING EXERCISES

Once you've loosened and lengthened your muscles sufficiently, it's time to begin to strengthen them. A strong core is a healthy core and is your best bet to help prevent further pelvic floor dysfunction in the future.

Strengthening isn't just about getting hard muscles, either. Strength affects several aspects of your overall health. Strong muscles improve your posture, and a body that is better aligned works better. Moreover, strong muscles assist in healthy circulation. Your metabolism is increased, your system—including your digestive system—works more efficiently, and toned muscles make you feel better emotionally and may increase your confidence. So the four exercises you'll do in this part are an important step toward your general well-being as well as toward a healthier pelvic floor.

It's important to note that you'll be *adding* these exercises to the Letting Go exercises of Part 1, not replacing anything. In fact, you can make these next four exercises a part of your cardio routine.

But the four are aimed specifically at easing your pain by strengthening your core. Start with five repetitions of each exercise, and as your symptoms improve and the exercises get easier—probably in a month or two—work your way up to 30 reps of each. When the 30 reps become as easy as a walk in the park, you can add weights or try some other techniques for making the exercises more challenging. I'll offer recommendations for how to do that at the end of each section.

For now, however, keep it simple, and take it easy as you begin the exercises to strengthen your core. Remember that if you start Part 2 and you find that your symptoms are back, you have probably moved too quickly to the Part 2 exercises. It happens frequently: you start to feel better, and you're so eager to move on that you do so before you're fully ready. If that happens, don't be discouraged; just go back to Part 1, get those symptoms well improved, then move on to Part 2.

Don't forget to breathe while exercising.

Step 1: Tight Abs

The transverse abdominus is a muscle deep in the abdomen that wraps around your lower abdomen above your pelvis, like a corset. In strengthening the transverse abdominus, you also help to stabilize your core. Here's how.

1. Lie on your back, bend your legs at the knee with the knees hip-width apart, and make sure both feet are flat on the floor.

2. As if you were zipping up a tight pair of jeans, tighten your navel down toward your spine, keeping your spine in a neutral position. Don't "suck in" your belly; just contract it so that you feel the muscles in your lower abdomen tighten. Do not tilt your pelvis up or down. Do not bear down on or tighten the pelvic floor muscles. All of that is counterproductive to what this exercise sets out to do.
3. Hold the contraction for five seconds, relax for five seconds, then repeat for the full five repetitions.
4. Over time, increase the hold to 10 seconds with 5 seconds of relaxation between reps.

Advanced Version. There are two ways to make this exercise more challenging and more fun.

- Add a head lift. Place both hands gently behind your head and lift your head about 12 inches, making sure to keep your chin tucked in. Start by doing 25 basic tight abs exercises and five with head lifts. Then gradually increase to 30 with head lifts.

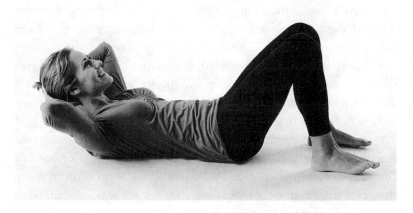

- Add a knee lift. While keeping your abs tight, slowly lift one foot about 20 inches and lower. Switch legs. Again, start by doing five of these in addition to 25 basic tight abs moves, then gradually increase to 30 with knee lift.

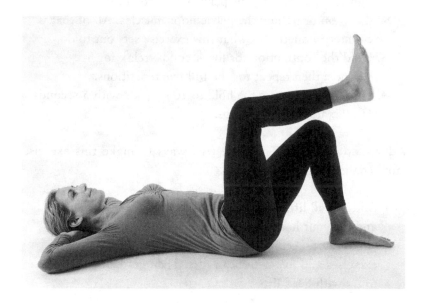

One important caution before you undertake the abdominal exercises: if you have diastisis recti, you will need to perform a corrective exercise first. Diastisis recti is a fairly common disorder in which the right and left muscles of the abdomen, specifically the rectus abdominus, which are attached to one another with connective tissue, have become separated. Common causes of the separation are chronic straining, pregnancy, obesity, and more. To test for diastisis recti, lie down on your back, knees bent, feet on the floor or bed. Place two fingers about an inch directly below the navel and lift your head to contract the abdominal muscles. Then place two fingers about an inch directly above the navel and lift your head to contract the abdominal muscles. If you feel a separation of more than two fingers in either location, chances are you have diastisis recti, in which case I recommend you see a physical therapist or healthcare provider for a proper diagnosis.

Step 2: Bridge

The bridge exercise targets your quadriceps muscles on the top of your thighs, your hamstrings, your lower back and abdomen, and the gluteal muscles of your butt. But take care: if you have pain when you sit, or if your pain symptoms increase when doing this exercise, stop! Move on to the next exercise in the routine.

You can count out the bridge in sequences of seconds: three, three, three, and five.

1. Lie on your back with both knees bent, hip-width apart, and with both feet flat on the floor. Your arms should be alongside your body. As in Step 1, tight abs, tighten your transverse abdominus muscle.

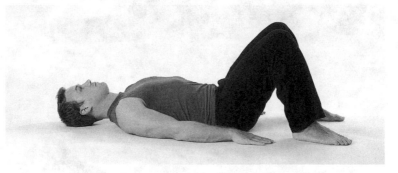

2. Take three seconds to slowly raise your pelvis.
3. When you reach the top of the "bridge," hold the position for three seconds.

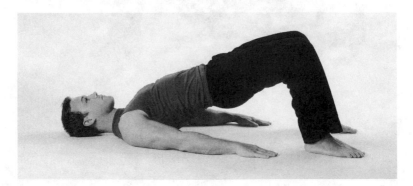

4. Lower slowly for a count of three seconds.

5. Back at the starting position, relax everything for five seconds, then repeat for the full five repetitions.

Advanced Version. Try doing a one-legged bridge. Start with the basic position, then straighten one leg. Tighten the abdominals and keep your pelvis square as you raise your buttocks off the ground with one leg. Repeat five times on one side and five on the other. Slowly increase the reps as the exercise gets easier.

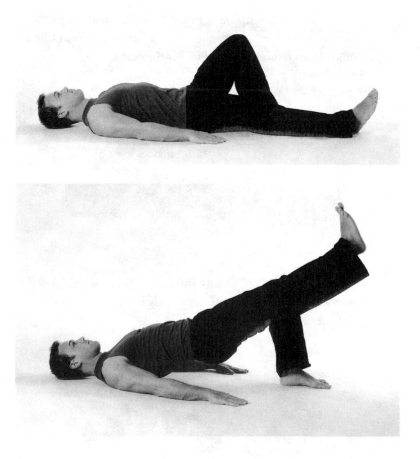

Step 3: Quadruped—Opposite Arm and Leg Raise

For this exercise, we go back to prehistoric times before we humans stood upright. If it hurts to sit or if you have tightness in the gluteal muscles of your butt, only do the arm portion of this exercise. Otherwise, this down-on-all-fours exercise strengthens your back, shoulder muscles, gluteal muscles, hamstrings, and abdominal muscles. (If you find you cannot lift the opposite arm and leg simultaneously, start by lifting the arm and leg separately, holding each for three seconds, until you can manage to raise both at the same time.)

1. Get down on all fours on your hands and knees. Hold your head in a straight line with your spine, with your chin tucked in.

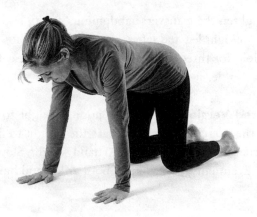

2. Keeping your back and neck straight, tighten your navel up to your spine, contracting your transverse abdominus muscle just as you did in the tight abs exercise. It may help to imagine that there is a pole resting on your back and you have to make sure it doesn't roll off.

3. Still holding the abdominal muscle tight, lift your left leg and right arm simultaneously while keeping your pelvis square to the floor. Hold for three seconds, then lower both arm and leg. Relax.

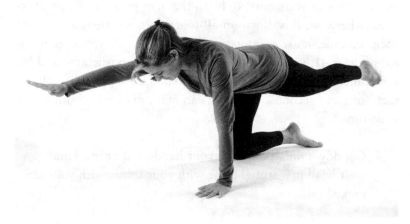

4. Tighten the transverse abdominus again, and now raise your right leg and left arm.
5. Hold for three seconds, lower, relax. Repeat five times on each side.

Advanced Version. Add a half-pound weight to your ankle as you do the exercise. Slowly increase the weight to five pounds.

Alternatively, add a half-pound hand weight. Slowly increase the weight. Eventually, you can add both ankle and hand weights.

Step 4: Squats

Not to be attempted by anyone with knee problems (except under the guidance of a trained professional), squats can nevertheless strengthen the abdominals, quads, hamstrings, lower back, and glutes. The important thing to remember, however, is that your knees should not extend beyond your toes. Here's the right way to do squats:

1. Stand with feet hip-width apart and feet slightly forward of the line of your shoulders, toes turned slightly out. Tighten your abs.

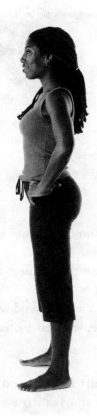

2. Slowly, on a count of three seconds, bend your knees as you lower your buttocks to a maximum of a 45-degree angle—or as close as possible. Lean forward slightly as you do this, but keep your back straight. The action is what you would do if you were about to sit down on a chair. Look carefully at the photo to see what I mean.

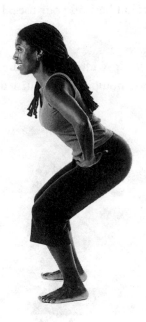

3. Rise back up to a standing position, also on a three-second count.
4. Relax for five seconds, and repeat five times.

Advanced Version. Hold a one-pound weight in each hand for the full 30 reps. In due course, you may increase the amount of weight.

Part 2 Schedule
Add Part 2 exercises to Part 1 routine: do daily in conjunction with your cardio routine, and slowly increase the reps of each exercise to 30.

PART 3: GET ACTIVE

Your own body is the best judge of when you should resume your favorite recreational activities. When the pain has diminished, when you're feeling strong enough, when both the Letting Go and the strengthening exercises, including your cardio exercise activity, have become second nature, that's when you should think about going back to your preferred sport.

But whenever you do so, the key is to *ease into it*. And the warning is that if you don't, you can not only undo the good you've done, but you may actually set yourself back even further. So whatever the activity is, start off slowly and lightly, work your way up, level by level, take plenty of breaks, and don't tire yourself out. Fatigue is a fast route to injury.

The key is to monitor yourself and your pain as you return to the activity, and to think of your return as occurring in three parts, as follows:

- **Beginner Part 3.** Start out doing one-tenth of what you would "normally" do—a tenth as much as you used to do before your pain or discomfort made the activity no fun at all. Go at one-tenth the speed, do one-tenth the distance, spend one-tenth the time. If your typical hike was five miles, start out with a half-mile trek. Instead of a full day on the slopes, start with two hours, and stick to the easier slopes.
- **Intermediate Part 3.** Slowly increase the variables by a tenth. *Slowly.* Take two weeks' worth of half-mile hikes before you try a walk of a mile. Spend two weeks skiing for two hours a day only before you add the third hour. Yes, this seems slow, and you may find it frustrating, but surely a little frustration is worth it to avoid the backsliding that can happen so quickly if you overdo your return to activity.
- **Advanced Part 3.** Finally, when you have incrementally worked your way back to your full capacity, practice performing at full capacity *for short intervals only*, making sure to take plenty of breaks. That means that instead of taking on a tennis match against the kid with the killer serve, bat the ball around with a friend for a set or two, a friend who will understand that you might have to quit

playing suddenly—best of all, a friend who might remind you that you need to pay attention to your body, watch for negative symptoms, and take it easy.

Keep in mind that you may not feel the increased pelvic pain for a day or two—which is all the more reason to take it slowly. All of this pretty much means that team sports are out for now. When teammates are relying on you, you feel you have to give your all, and giving your all right now is just about the last thing you need to do. So stay on the sidelines, practice your sport as an individual, and wait till you can give it everything you've got before you re-up as a starter.

That still leaves you lots of leeway for sports and recreational activity.

Is Rollerblading your thing? Start off with a short, easy ride on a level surface in a nearby park. Aim for just getting back the feel of being on skates, not for speed.

Maybe you're a hiker. If so, get back into hiking by taking a little walk in the woods carrying a lightweight pack. Don't start off with a four-day trek into mountainous wilderness, even if that was the last thing you did before your pain or disorder made it impossible to do anything at all.

Yoga is your preferred form of exercise? Just because it's famous for being a healthy way to increase flexibility doesn't mean that the twisting called for in some of its postures won't send you back to square one. Be gentle with yourself, and if you feel any pain at all, stop! Start off with restorative yoga, and slowly work your way up to the more advanced practices.

If you're a skier, stay off the black diamond trail for the present. You may not need to go back to the bunny slope, but think about starting off on a flat blue trail this season.

After all, the one thing worse than going back to basics in your favorite sport or recreational activity would be going back to the incapacitating pain that made you stop the activity in the first place. It bears repeating: for your return to sports and recreation, ease into it. Take it slowly, and be careful.

KEEPING THE EXERCISES CHALLENGING

Although it's essential to start any exercise program slowly and modestly, it's equally essential to build up to a point where the exercises are doing you the most good. But how do you know when to move to the next step?

Here's a simple formula: When the last three repetitions have become easy, you're ready to add another five. That means if you have started with five reps of an exercise, and after a week or so, reps 3–5 are a piece of cake—and assuming always that there is no increase in pain or other symptoms—start doing 10 reps. When you've been doing 10 for a while and reps 8–10 have become a breeze, move up to 15.

If you need the strengthening exercises to be more difficult, go back and add the advanced exercises to your routine. For purposes of this toning program, I'm not recommending that you go beyond 30 repetitions of any exercise.

If eventually you find that 30 reps of each exercise, even with challenging variations and weights added, is just too easy, you are probably ready to move to another level of exercise—providing, of course, that you are symptom-free. In that case, consult with a licensed physical therapist or exercise physiologist so you can be sure you're not undertaking anything that could injure what you've spent all this time and effort healing.

RECAP: THE END-THE-PAIN ROUTINE

Part 1: Letting Go Exercises

Step 1: Breathe   Inhale for 3–5 seconds, exhale
                                for 4–6 seconds.
                                Do 5 reps, repeat throughout
                                the day.

Step 2: Drop

Inhale for 3–5 seconds.
Visualize the "release" on
    exhale for 4–6 seconds.
Do 5 reps, repeat throughout
    the day.

Step 3: Thigh Press

Hold 5 seconds.
Do 5 reps 2–4 times a day.

Step 4: Pelvic Floor Stretch

Hold 30–60 seconds.
Do 3 reps 2–4 times a day.

Step 5: Hip Rotator Stretch

Hold 30–60 seconds.
Do 3 reps 2–4 times a day.

Step 6: Hip Flexor Stretch

Hold 30–60 seconds each side.
Do 3 reps 2–4 times a day.

Step 7: Abdominals Stretch

Hold 30–60 seconds.
Do 3 reps 2–4 times a day.

Step 8: Back Stretch

Hold 30–60 seconds.
Do 3 reps 2–4 times a day.

Step 9: Hamstrings Stretch

Hold 30–60 seconds.
Do 3 reps 2–4 times a day.

Step 10: Inner Thighs Stretch

Hold 30–60 seconds.
Do 3 reps 2–4 times a day.

Step 11: Butt Stretch

Hold 30–60 seconds.
Do 3 reps 2–4 times a day.

Part 2: Strengthening Exercises

Step 1: Tight Abs	Do 5–30 reps daily. Advanced version: Add head lift and/or knee lift.
Step 2: Bridge	Do 5–30 reps daily. Advanced version: One-legged bridge.
Step 3: Quadruped	Do 5–30 reps daily. Advanced version: Add weights.
Step 4: Squats	Do 5–30 reps daily. Advanced version: Add weights.

CHAPTER 4

STRENGTHEN THE MUSCLES

Do this program of exercises if you are suffering either bladder or bowel incontinence—or both—as a result of pelvic floor muscle weakness or pelvic organ prolapse, or if you have a feeling of heaviness or a falling-out feeling in the pelvic region with no accompanying pain. These exercises may also mitigate a decreased libido or an inability to achieve orgasm; men who suffer erectile dysfunction due to weak muscles may also benefit from these exercises. Do not do them if you feel any urgency, pain, constipation, or retention, if you must relieve yourself frequently at night, or if you have any of the symptoms described in Chapter 3. You must wait until those symptoms are 100 percent improved through the End-the-Pain routine before you undertake them. Only then should you begin to slowly integrate these exercises into your normal daily routine. If the previous symptoms return, stop these exercises and return to the End-the-Pain routine only. Symptoms indicating the use of these exercises may include the following:

In Both Men and Women
- Stress urinary or bowel incontinence (involuntary leakage due to an increase in abdominal pressure, as from sneezing, coughing, running, etc.)

- Pelvic organ prolapse
- Decreased libido due to weak pelvic floor muscles
- Difficulty achieving orgasm due to weak pelvic floor muscles

In Women Only
- Prenatal and postpartum stress incontinence
- Cystocele (descent of anterior vaginal wall)
- Rectocele (descent of posterior vaginal wall)
- Enterocele (descent of intestine)
- Uterocele (descent of the uterus)
- Urethrocele (descent of the urethra)

In Men Only
- Erectile dysfunction
- Rectal organ prolapse

Incontinence is the involuntary leaking of urine, feces, or gas. Often, people only become aware of the problem when they note staining on their underclothing.

But incontinence is really just a symptom. It signals a weakness in the muscles of the pelvic floor. Strengthen those muscles, and you very likely will end the incontinence.

How do the muscles of the pelvic floor grow weak? There are any number of possible causes. Childbirth can certainly weaken the pelvic floor. So can surgery; for example, we frequently see this muscle weakness and the resulting incontinence in men who have undergone prostatectomy for the treatment of prostate cancer. Injury or trauma, an illness that decreases the immune system, fatigue, or hormonal changes can also diminish the strength and elasticity of these muscles. If you lift heavy weights all day long and are straining your pelvic floor muscles as you do so, if you're excessively overweight or obese, if you have very poor posture, if you find yourself straining against a condition of constipation, you can weaken your pelvic floor. And, unfortunately, these muscles also lose strength as we age and grow less active.

And while incontinence is perhaps the most evident of the symptoms of this weakness, there are others. One is organ prolapse—when a part of the bladder or another organ literally slips out of place, producing a feeling of fullness as if something is falling out of you. Prolapse happens when the muscles and connective tissue have become so weak they are no longer holding up the organ; with no "floor" to support it, the organ simply sags.

Sex is another area where muscle weakness can be telling: individuals may have difficulty achieving orgasm when the pelvic floor muscles are weak, for those are the muscles that work to increase blood flow, stimulation, and satisfaction.

Clearly, the way to address all these symptoms is to strengthen the muscles of the pelvic floor, and that's just what the Strengthen-the-Muscles routine sets out to do. It proceeds in four parts. The key to all the parts of the Strengthen-the-Muscles program is the Kegel exercise you'll learn in Part 1. But perhaps just as important as learning to do Kegels correctly is to learn to relax the pelvic floor muscles between exercises.

RELAXING THE PELVIC FLOOR TO STRENGTHEN IT

One of my first patients many years ago was a Pilates instructor—I'll call her Sandy. As I'm sure you know, Pilates is a wonderful program of exercises geared precisely to enhancing core strength and flexibility. Sandy, in her mid-50s, was a sweet and delightful woman who was a living example of Pilates' strengths.

So I was surprised that she had come to my physical therapy studio complaining of a gradual onset of urinary urgency and frequency along with difficulty achieving orgasm. The urinary urgency had recently developed into urinary urge incontinence—that is, Sandy would feel a strong urge, would rush to the bathroom, but would invariably end up leaking before she got there.

Both Sandy and I were puzzled that a Pilates practitioner, who regularly worked the muscles of her core, could have a weak pelvic floor. In fact, on that first visit, Sandy enthusiastically demonstrated for me some of her Pilates teaching. She lay on her back, engaged her abdominals, and lifted her pelvic floor muscles as she slowly raised one leg and smoothly did leg circles in the air. She switched legs. She showed me the signature Pilates 100, challenging the abs and back. All the while, Sandy kept repeating what she told her students during a teaching session: "And, tighten those abdominal muscles and *lift* the pelvic floor. And tighten. And lift. Tighten. And lift."

Watching and listening, I suddenly had an insight into what the problem was. "Sandy," I asked her, "do you ever have your class *relax* the pelvic floor—or are you always tightening and never resting those muscles?" She replied that since the aim was to keep the students' heart rate relatively high during class, she limited the resting to three times during the one-hour session.

I was pretty sure that was the key to the diagnosis of Sandy's problem. "By resting so rarely," I suggested, "you're never really relaxing the pelvic floor muscles. The result is that they have probably shortened and are now pulling on your bladder and urethra, and that's what's causing your urinary urgency and frequency. Moreover," I explained, "shortened pelvic floor muscles have a difficult time contracting and going through their full range of motion. That's why you're having trouble coming to orgasm and with leaking."

The answer, I suggested, was to reeducate Sandy's pelvic floor muscles to relax—basically, to do the End-the-Pain routine of Chapter 3. For although in her case the muscles were probably not weak, their inability to relax certainly diminished their power—with the resulting incontinence and sexual dysfunction.

The bottom line? Relaxing the muscles between exercises is as important as the exercises themselves. Your muscles won't function with strength unless you learn how to relax them, so be sure to follow carefully the instructions to relax the muscles in these exercises. In addition, it's a good idea to relax altogether between each set of exercises.

Also, don't forget to breathe. As you learned in the End-the-Pain routine, not breathing—holding your breath—while you exercise is completely counterproductive. Breathe deeply before each exercise, then start to count as you begin the exercise—whatever it is. This forces you to breathe while doing the exercise. After a while, this becomes automatic.

So take a breath, and let's begin those exercises now.

Part 1: Your Strength Foundation—Doing Your Kegels, Tightening Your Abs (2 Weeks)

10-second slow Kegels	10 reps 3 times a day
2-second fast Kegels	10 reps 3 times a day
Tight abs	10–30 reps, once a day

Part 2: Intermediate Exercises—Hips, Bridge, Tilt with Kegels (4 Weeks)

Hip external rotation	10–30 reps, once a day
Hip adduction	10–30 reps, once a day
Bridge	10–30 reps, once a day
Pelvic tilt	10–30 reps, once a day

Part 3: Challenging Exercises—Standing Kegels (4 Weeks)

Slow standing Kegels	5–10 reps, once a day
Fast standing Kegels	5–10 reps, once a day
One-foot squat with Kegel	5–10 reps, once a day
Two-foot squat with Kegel	5–10 reps, once a day
Sit-and-stand with Kegel	5–10 reps, once a day

Part 4: Advanced Exercises—Action Kegels (4 Weeks)

Marching in place	10 reps, once a day
Small jumps	10 reps, once a day
Big jumps	10 reps, once a day
Lunges	10 reps, once a day

PART I: YOUR STRENGTH FOUNDATION—DOING YOUR KEGELS, TIGHTENING YOUR ABS

Dr. Arnold Kegel, who died in 1981, was a Los Angeles–based gynecologist who developed exercises for regularly clenching and unclenching the muscles of the pelvic floor. Kegel developed the exercises to help his patients increase their sexual function and gratification as well as to address problems of prolapse and incontinence. Although the exercises now bear his name—we tell patients to "Do your Kegels"—the methodology has really been known since ancient times and has numerous variants in the practices of Eastern religions.

Kegels are what are called resistive exercises. Specifically, as you deliberately control a muscle's movement, you incrementally increase its ability to contract. As you do your Kegels over time, this contractile strength will grow, and the muscles of your pelvic floor will become broader and thicker and will gain increased muscle tone.

But not everybody should do Kegels. If you find that the Kegel clench causes pain or increased bladder or bowel frequency or urgency, stop. It may mean that the pelvic floor muscles are spasmed or shortened, and doing the Kegels may only spasm or shorten them further. See your doctor or health-care provider if that is the case. Also, it's advisable to consult with a gynecologist or a pelvic floor physical therapist to make sure that your incontinence problem is in fact a result of a weakened pelvic floor or possible prolapsed organ. In other words, be sure of the cause before you attempt Kegels as the solution.

The Strengthen-the-Muscles routine calls for doing Kegels in conjunction with an exercise for tightening your core abdominal muscle, the transverse abdominus. Although they are only connected by fascia (connective tissue), these two sets of muscles deep in the body's core—the pelvic floor and the transverse abdominus—are mutually supportive. They need to work together, and for that to happen with maximum benefit, they also need to be equally fit. That's why Part 1 of the Strengthen-the-Muscles routine asks you to strengthen both by doing the Kegel and tight abs exercises as a pair.

Start, however, by doing the two exercises separately—maybe doing your Kegels in the morning and tight abs at night. Once you're comfortable doing both, by all means put the two together. This will not only enhance your core strength and coordination, it will also decrease the time spent on your exercise routine by some five minutes.

Their joint effect is beneficial in many ways. Obviously, these exercises enhance muscle strength, and they increase the flow of blood to the muscles and the pelvic organs as well. The risk of infection is thereby lowered, and that too helps stave off pelvic floor disorders. What's more, the strengthening of these muscles can enhance sexual stimulation and sexual gratification as well.

Spend at least two weeks on Part 1.

Kegels: Find the Muscles

Kegels are absolutely basic to the entire Strengthen-the-Muscles routine, and it's very important that they be done correctly. Done wrong, Kegels simply won't work, and patients who don't see results can grow discouraged. Even worse, you could end up with more problems. For example, if you do the Kegels wrong and instead are overusing accessory muscles like the glutes or the inner thighs, this could produce trigger points on those muscles—that is, hyperirritable spots that are painful to the touch and that can also lead to new pain and new problems.

The key to doing Kegels correctly is to locate your own pelvic floor muscles. There's a simple way to do this: while urinating, stop the urine from flowing by tightening or squeezing the muscles. Those are the muscles you're going to clench and unclench when you do your Kegels. If you find that clenching the muscles minimizes but does not completely stop the urine stream, you've found the right muscles, but you've also learned that they're very weak indeed—a solid indication that you need to do the Strengthen-the-Muscles routine.

Do this locating and identifying exercise very briefly and only temporarily—maybe once a week initially, until you identify the muscles—because doing it repeatedly while urinating sends a confusing signal to the brain that may eventually produce a urinary dysfunction.

Another way to locate the muscles you're looking for is during sexual activity. Squeeze around your partner's finger or penis; the muscle you tighten in doing so is the precise muscle you'll want to clench and unclench—contract and relax—when you do your Kegels.

Step 1: The Kegel Exercise

Here's how to do your Kegels to strengthen your pelvic floor:

Lie or sit down, whichever you prefer. You may use a pillow as a wedge under the small of your back if you like.

Find the muscle you identified earlier and clench it, then relax. Clench again, then relax. And so on. One clench-and-relax constitutes a repetition, and both sides of the repetition—both the clenching and the unclenching—are equally important. Remember Sandy, the Pilates instructor? Relax as deliberately and for as long as you clench the muscle.

You may find it difficult to do Kegels at first if your muscles are very weak. But each repetition really will increase the strength of the muscles, and in time, doing your Kegels will become easier—guaranteed. Do these Kegels three times a day if you have one of the problems listed at the beginning of this chapter, but *no more than three times a week* if you're doing them just to enhance your sex life.

Here's the formula:

1. Tighten the muscle and hold for 10 seconds, relax for 10 seconds. Do 10 repetitions to strengthen your slow-twitch pelvic floor muscles.
2. Tighten and hold for two seconds, relax for two seconds. Do 10 repetitions to strengthen the fast-twitch fiber muscles.

The two different basic Kegel exercises differ only in timing, not in the process. What's the difference?

Your first set of Kegels, held for 10 seconds, then relaxed for 10, addresses the slow-twitch fibers that make up some 70 percent of the muscles. These are the muscle fibers that provide support and resist fatigue. The second set of Kegels—two-second Kegels—strengthen those fast-contraction fibers that help open and close the bladder and bowel and that are so essential in sexual activity. The two sets of Kegels mean you're strengthening both your marathon endurance muscles and the sprinter muscles that provide a quick jolt of power when needed.

Step 2: Tight Abs

If you've done the End-the-Pain routine, you already know about the tight abs exercise. It's an exercise for strengthening the muscle known as the transverse abdominus, the muscle deep in the abdomen that wraps around your lower abdomen above your pelvis, like a corset. In strengthening the transverse abdominus, you also help to stabilize your core. Do the exercise once a day:

1. Lie on your back, bend your legs at the knee with knees hip-width apart, and make sure both feet are flat on the floor.

2. As if you were zipping up a tight pair of jeans, tighten your navel down toward your spine, keeping your spine in a neutral position. Don't "suck in" your belly; just contract it so that you feel the muscles in your lower abdomen tighten. Do not tilt your pelvis up or down. Do not bear down on the pelvic floor muscles. All of that is counterproductive to what this exercise sets out to do.

3. Hold the contraction for five seconds, relax for five seconds. Do five repetitions. Over time, increase the hold to 10 seconds with five seconds of relaxation between reps, and increase the repetitions to 30.

PART 2: INTERMEDIATE EXERCISES— HIPS, BRIDGE, TILT

Once you have been doing Kegels and the tight abs exercise successfully for a couple of weeks, you're ready to add hip and additional core exercises to the basic Strengthen-the-Muscles routine. The muscles of the hips and core all work together with one another and with the pelvic floor and assist in stabilizing the pelvis, the abdomen, and the back. Take another look at the diagram of the pelvis in Chapter 1 (Figures 1.1 and 1.2), and you will see again how all these muscles form that bowl-like sling at the body's core. Weakness in these muscles of the sling may result in dysfunction in the low part of the back, the pelvis, and the sacroiliac region, and it may also lead to incontinence and prolapsed pelvic organs.

That's why we add the following four exercises to the Strengthen-the-Muscles routine. The idea is do a Kegel contract-and-relax while you do each of these exercises. That takes concentration and may be difficult at first. If so, get comfortable with the exercises of Part 2 on their own to begin with, then add the Kegels later on.

If you manage to do all four of the Part 2 exercises with Kegels—in other words, you are able to do the hip external rotation, hip adduction, bridge, and pelvic tilt while doing Kegels—Part 2 can simply replace the basic Kegels of Part 1. Otherwise, do at least two of these exercises every day in addition to your Kegels.

Whatever the number of Part 2 exercises you do, it's very important to do them slowly and with maximum control. If you toss them off quickly, you'll get no benefit at all. You might even injure yourself. So do each exercise slowly and deliberately. Concentrate.

For all four, you will be lying on your back with your knees bent. If you like, place a thin pillow under your head for comfort.

Take four weeks to perfect Part 2.

Step 1: Hip External Rotation

On your back with your knees bent and feet together, tighten your transverse abdominus and slowly separate your knees—feet still together—until the knees are about 24 inches apart. Hold the position—with a Kegel—for three seconds, then slowly return your knees together in the center. Relax for five seconds.

Once this exercise becomes easy, you may add resistance by pressing your hands against the separation of the knees on the

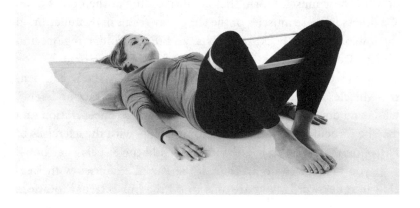

outside of your thighs. You may also use a resistance band for this purpose.

The hip external rotation exercise strengthens some of your butt muscles as well as your hip muscles. Do 10 repetitions, working up to 30 repetitions, once a day.

Step 2: Hip Adduction

You'll need a pillow or a ball for this exercise. On your back with your knees bent and feet hip-width apart, tighten your transverse abdominus, then squeeze the pillow or ball between your knees—while doing a Kegel—and hold the position for 10 seconds. Relax for 10 seconds. Do 10 repetitions of this inner thigh-strengthening exercise, increasing to 30 reps, once a day.

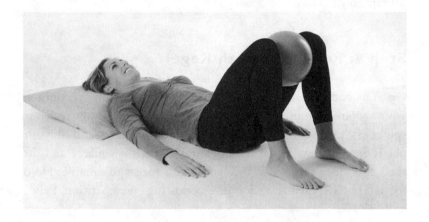

Step 3: Bridge

On your back, knees bent, feet flat and hip-width apart, tighten your transverse abdominus, then slowly raise your pelvis while doing a Kegel. Keep holding the muscles until you reach the top of

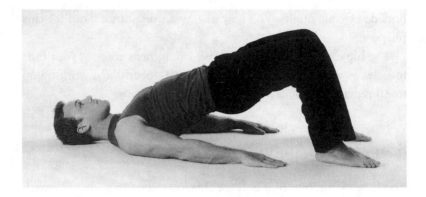

the bridge, then slowly lower the pelvis, still tightening the pelvic floor muscles.

Now relax totally for five seconds.

This exercise strengthens the top of the thigh, hamstrings, lower back, abs, and glutes. Repeat it a total of 10 times, increasing to 30 reps, once a day.

Step 4: Pelvic Tilt with Kegel

On your back, knees bent, feet flat and hip-width apart, tighten your abdominal muscles by sinking your belly button toward your spine—as if you were zipping up a tight pair of jeans—and tilt your pelvis upward toward the ceiling. Simultaneously, squeeze and lift the pelvic floor muscles in a Kegel. Don't forget to breathe. Hold for 10 seconds, then relax for 10 seconds for one repetition. Pelvic

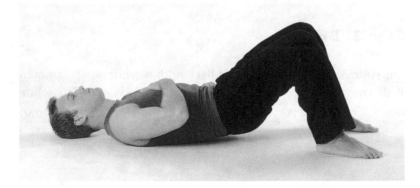

tilts strengthen your abdominal muscles and help to stabilize your core. Do 10 repetitions, increasing to 30 reps, once a day.

As I explained in Chapter 3—and it bears repeating here—there is one important caution before you undertake the abdominal exercises: if you have diastisis recti, you will need to perform a corrective exercise first. Diastisis recti is a fairly common disorder in which the right and left muscles of the abdomen, which are attached to one another with connective tissue, have become separated. Common causes of the separation are chronic straining, pregnancy, obesity, and more. To test for diastisis recti, lie down on your back, knees bent, feet on the floor or bed. Place two fingers about an inch directly below the navel and lift your head to contract the abdominal muscles. Then place two fingers about an inch directly above the navel and lift your head to contract the abdominal muscles. If you feel a separation of more than two fingers in either location, chances are you have diastisis recti, in which case I recommend you see a physical therapist or healthcare provider for a proper diagnosis.

PART 3: CHALLENGING EXERCISES— STANDING KEGELS

When you stand upright, your pelvic floor muscles are parallel to the floor and are thus fighting gravity. The three exercises of Part 3, therefore, provide a particular challenge to your muscles—especially since you must do a Kegel simultaneously with each exercise. Again, do each exercise slowly and in a controlled manner in order to avoid injury and gain maximum benefit for your effort. Take four weeks for Part 3.

Step 1: The Standing Kegel

Stand with your feet hip-width apart. Do five slow Kegels as you breathe deeply: hold for 10 seconds, rest for 10 seconds. Then do five fast Kegels: hold for two seconds, rest for two seconds. Work up to 10 repetitions of both the 10-second and two-second standing Kegels.

Step 2: One-Foot Squat with Kegel

Start with feet a foot apart as you contract your abdominal muscles and tighten your pelvic floor in a Kegel. Now, with your back straight, slowly lower your buttocks and bend your knees to 45 degrees, making sure the knees do not extend past the toes. Hold for three seconds, then rise up slowly, still maintaining the Kegel. Now relax for three seconds.

Do five repetitions, and slowly work up to 10. Once you have worked up to 10 reps, you are ready to advance to the two-foot squat with Kegel (Step 3).

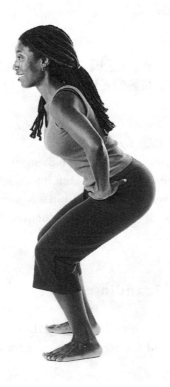

Step 3: Two-Foot Squat with Kegel

Do exactly the same thing as in the previous exercise, but squat with your feet two feet apart. Start with five reps, and work up to 10.

Step 4: Sit-and-Stand

You'll need a firm chair without wheels. Start out seated at the edge of the chair with your feet hip-width apart, flat on the floor, and slightly back so you have leverage to stand. Keeping your back straight, lean forward at the hips, tighten your abdominal and pelvic floor muscles, and count to five as you slowly lift your buttocks off the chair and stand up. Rest, standing, for three seconds. With knees still hip-width apart and with your back straight, tighten your abdominals, do a Kegel, and count to five as you slowly lower yourself back onto the chair; be careful not to extend your knees out beyond your toes. Do not flop onto the chair; that will defeat the muscle-strengthening purpose of the exercise.

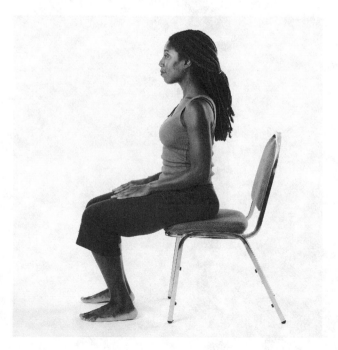

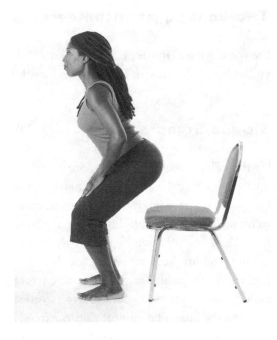

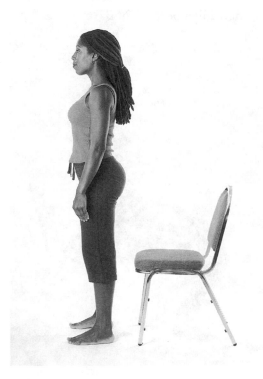

From seated position to seated position is one repetition. Start out doing five, and slowly work up to 10 repetitions. Don't forget to breathe!

If you find it too difficult to rise up out of the chair, try putting a couple of phone books on the seat. Gradually remove the books as you get stronger.

PART 4: ADVANCED EXERCISES— ACTION KEGELS

Although you'll be on the move for these exercises, it's still important to do them slowly, while breathing, and in a controlled manner. Also, you must do a Kegel with each exercise, so you'll need to concentrate.

Step 1: Marching in Place

Tighten your abs and do a Kegel as you march in place for 10 seconds. Rest for five seconds. Do this 10 times. To make it more challenging, lift your knees higher and march faster, making sure that you maintain tight abs and tightened pelvic floor muscles for the full 10 seconds.

Step 2: Small Jumps

Tighten your abs and do a Kegel as you jump one to two inches off the ground. Rest for two seconds. Do 10 repetitions.

Step 3: Big Jumps

Tighten your abs and do a Kegel and jump up five to six inches. Take a two-second rest. Do 10 of these big jumps.

Step 4: Lunges

Stand with feet hip-width apart. Keeping your torso upright and your pelvis square, extend your right foot three feet in front of your left foot. Tighten your abs and your pelvic floor muscles in a Kegel, and slowly lower your torso straight down so that your left knee bends between 45 and 90 degrees—depending on your strength and comfort level. Hold this lunge position for three seconds. Still holding the tight abs and Kegel, and with torso still upright, slowly raise yourself as you straighten your right knee. Rest for five seconds.

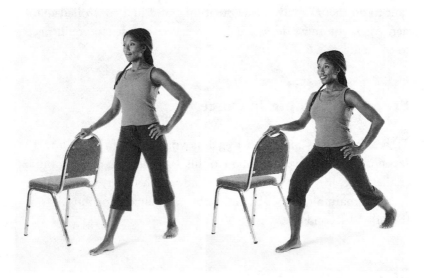

Do 10 repetitions, then switch legs, extending your left foot in front of your right. Do the exercise 10 more times with the left foot in front.

RECAP: THE STRENGTHEN-THE-MUSCLES EXERCISE ROUTINE

As you gain the muscular strength you're seeking in these exercises, you can adjust the routine. At first, Kegels, which are basic to the Strengthen-the-Muscles routine, can easily be incorporated into your daily activities. Do them when you find yourself listening to a presentation at work, or at the movies, or while commuting on the bus or train. Or, as I mentioned earlier, if you are able to integrate Kegels into Parts 2 through 4, then you need not do the exercises of Part 1.

Once you've advanced through the total three-and-a-half month program and have gained proficiency and comfort in each part—as well as enhanced muscle strength—you can consolidate your daily workout into a minimum of five exercises, choosing any you like from Parts 2, 3, and 4. Be sure to vary the five—or more—exercises you do each day. Mix it up so that you continue to address all the components of the pelvic floor and keep yourself fit all over, inside and out.

Keep up Parts 2, 3 and 4 even if your symptoms have improved 100 percent—but at this point only three or four times a week. It is a good practice for a lifetime of well-being. If, however, your symptoms persist after three and a half months, see a specialist in pelvic floor dysfunction and incontinence.

CHAPTER 5

GIVE YOURSELF A MASSAGE

Everybody loves getting a massage.

Whether it's at an elegant seaside spa with ocean breezes wafting over your lotion-soaked body as sweet music plays, or on a utilitarian folding table in the local gym, getting a massage is a luxury. It relaxes us, makes us feel at peace, and sends our physical and emotional aches and pains packing.

But where your pelvic floor disorder is concerned, massage is also an essential tool of the healing process. The massages you'll learn in this chapter are not just about chilling out; they're about lengthening the muscles and tissues of your pelvic floor and the surrounding area, diminishing the points of irritation in the muscles, removing the toxins that cause tension in your body's tissue, and increasing the flow of blood.

Result? Your pain is reduced. And as we have seen, when the pain subsides, it can reverse the cascade of pelvic floor disorder and pain. Less pain means that the structures and organs of the body are able to function better, and that reduces the pain even further, which in turn helps the underlying structures and organs function still better, and so on. The bottom line is healing, and that's what this book is all about.

What's more, you can do these massages yourself. In the privacy of your own home. At your convenience. Although if you like, of course, there's nothing nicer than having your spouse or partner, a trained professional, or even a good friend do these massages for you.

One important caveat about massage: whether internal or external, massage may cause soreness or even bruising. This is natural. It's part of the healing. It's a signal that you need the massaging. But the soreness should last no longer than four days, after which you can return to massaging that area. If the soreness persists, see your health-care practitioner.

You'll learn two massages in this chapter. One addresses the tight spots—the sore points or trigger points, called this because they trigger pain—in your muscles and underlying tissues that contribute to your pelvic floor pain and other symptoms. As we've seen, pelvic floor pain can feel like it's happening all over, when actually it may be located in one or another specific area but radiating outward. With this simple massage, you'll find the sore points—one after another after another—and apply pressure to massage each spot. Believe it or not, done repeatedly over time, this will loosen your muscles, diminish the soreness, and alleviate the pain.

The sore points massage, as I call it, is an absolutely essential part of the natural way to heal your pelvic floor disorder. Do it in conjunction with the End-the-Pain routine you learned in Chapter 3; in fact, it's wise to begin every day with the sore points massage before you begin your exercise program.

The second self-massage you'll learn in this chapter works wonders if you are suffering the discomforts of bloating, constipation, or excessive gas. It's called the ILU massage—you'll see why when we get to it—and it can actually help mitigate the problem as well as soothe the discomfort. By the same token, if diarrhea is the issue, the ILU massage can calm your nervous gut and slow its contractions. Use this massage when you need it—or any time you just want to relax.

SELF-MASSAGING YOUR SORE POINTS

How do you get rid of the tight spots—the sore points—in your muscles and in the underlying tissue? Massage them out.

Sore points really are tight nodules in the muscle that have become "hyperirritable," as medical researchers put it. They are trigger points; touch them, and you feel pain, and the pain often shoots outward: it becomes radiating pain. This massage releases the tightness so that the pain subsides and the radiating distance shortens; eventually, the pain just goes away.

There are four areas that you'll address in doing the sore points massage: your thighs, the gluteal muscles of your butt, your abdomen, and your pelvic floor—both outside and inside. You don't need any special gizmos to do the sore points massage, although you may find it useful to use a tennis ball, rubber ball, or a massage tool—usually made of wood or hard rubber and available at some health food stores and pharmacies—for the external massages, and you may find it easier to use a dilator for the internal massage. But all you really need is a comfortable place to lie down, some solitude, and a few minutes of time.

Do the massage once a day, and concentrate each day on one of the four different areas of sore points—the thighs one day, the gluteal muscles of your backside on the second day, the abdominal muscles on the third day, and the pelvic floor muscles on the fourth day. On the fifth day, you start all over again with the thigh self-massage.

You may find it helpful to use a massage cream. You can find massage creams and oils at most drugstores and at some health food stores. Or use your favorite skin moisturizer. The key is to use very little of it—only as much as fits on a single fingertip. Rub it into your hands, and don't go back for more. The point is the pressure, not the cream.

Techniques for External Self-Massage

For the external massage of your thighs, glutes, and abdomen, there are two kinds of massage techniques you can use. Basically, you'll either press the pain away or roll it away. In both cases, you are helping to get rid of the trigger points and to lengthen the muscles and tissues that surround the pelvic floor, and that goes a long way toward healing.

The first technique, pressing (or kneading) the pain away, focuses on those trigger points I mentioned, and all you do is apply pressure and sustain it. Use your fingers to assess your pain, applying pressure gradually until you find the sore points. Then massage that point by holding pressure or by kneading the tissue for at least 30 and at most 90 seconds. That's really all there is to it. At first, the pressure may feel sharp, especially if the pain radiates outward, but as you continue to massage, the pain will subside and the radiating distance will diminish.

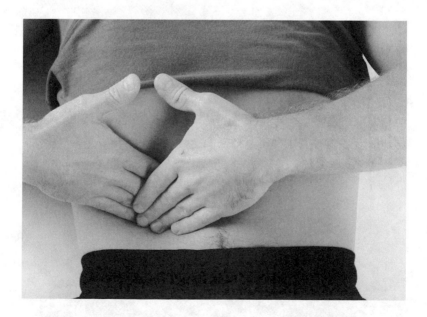

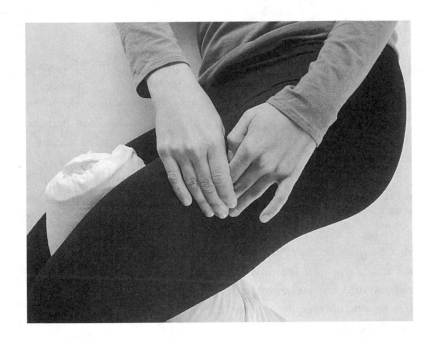

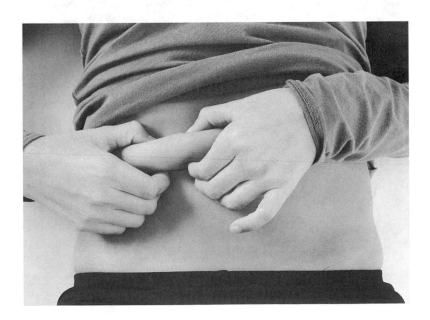

The second technique for massaging your sore points is with a kind of rolling technique: grab about an inch worth of skin and tissue with your fingers and thumb and try to move the skin like dough. It should move smoothly (see the bottom photograph on page 92). Use all your fingers and roll your skin in all different directions, feeling for the sore points and for tight tissue. Basically, what you're doing is mobilizing one layer of skin over the other in order to release the tension in the tissue. That helps increase the blood flow to the area and removes toxins from it, decreasing the pain and ultimately allowing more range of motion in the tissue and muscle.

As the pain decreases over time, gradually add pressure. If the pain should increase, stop the massage altogether.

Self-massage can be tiring, so do consider using a massage tool or vibrator on your sore points from time to time.

Here's what you do.

Thighs. Lie on your back with your knees bent up, feet flat. Place some pillows under your knees if you find that more comfortable. You can also lie on your side with a pillow between your knees, as shown in the top photograph on page 92. Using your index and middle finger or thumb, apply moderate pressure on the muscles of your inner thigh, outer thigh, front of thigh, and back of thigh—in that order. You're looking for a sore point—a spot in the muscle that feels taut or tight, that causes soreness when you touch it, or that repeats the pain or symptoms you're reading this book to heal. Basically, you'll know it when you feel it, and when you do, simply press down on or knead the sore point, or roll it around, for at least 30 and at most 90 seconds. Don't punch, poke, beat, or batter yourself. Just apply some pressure and hold it, or grab the skin and roll it. Then move on to the next sore point.

Gluteal Muscles. Do exactly the same thing with the gluteal muscle self-massage. Only this time, lie on your side with your knees bent and a pillow placed comfortably in between your knees. Reach around and press on various points on your backside, up, down, and across. When you sense tightness under your hand, or when you feel soreness or pain, apply pressure for 30 to 90 seconds, or grab and roll the connective tissue. Then move on until you find another sore point. When you've finished massaging the gluteal muscles you can easily reach on one side, turn onto your other side and repeat the procedure.

Abdomen. Lie on your back with your knees bent up, feet flat. Again, you can place pillows under your knees if you like. The area you're exploring here extends from the bottom of your rib cage all the way down to your pelvic bone, and from the sides of your core inward toward the belly button. Using your index and middle finger or thumb, apply moderate pressure on these muscles. Sustain the pressure when you locate a sore point, knead the underlying tissue, and/or roll the skin to loosen the tension, lengthen the muscle, and diminish the pain.

External and Internal Pelvic Floor Self-Massage

Although the self-massage principle is the same for this tender area of the body—find the sore points and apply pressure—the technique is far gentler, for the tissue and muscle here can be very sensitive. So do be good to yourself; remember that you are trying to soothe pain, not beat it into submission.

And obviously, be sure to wash your hands thoroughly with an antibacterial soap before and after you do any of the following massages. You may also use a non-latex glove, if that is more comfortable for you.

Let's start with the outside of the pelvic floor, an area called the perineal body, that portion of muscle and tissue located between the vaginal and anal areas in women and between the genitals and the anus in men. Refer to Figure 1.3, the female pelvic floor, or

1.4, the male pelvic floor, in Chapter 1. Lie back comfortably with your knees bent and feet flat. Apply a small amount of lubricant to the area; I recommend a natural lubricant that's paraben-free and has no propylene glycol, which can irritate the tissue. Then, gently apply pressure to the area for 30 to 90 seconds; this helps loosen the tissue and increase blood flow.

Note that this perineal massage is especially helpful before or after sexual activity. For women who may experience pain on penetration, this massage is useful prior to sexual activity. For both men and women, the perineal massage can minimize the tightening or spasming that inevitably occurs after orgasm. (Limit your sexual activity if it exacerbates your pain symptoms.)

Next come two forms of internal pelvic floor massage—the intravaginal for women and the intrarectal for both men and women. For women, the choice between the two is an issue of comfort: in some women, the vaginal tissue is so sensitive that they are more comfortable doing the massage rectally; others are uncomfortable doing a rectal massage and prefer the intravaginal version. Both forms, however, are useful to relax and lengthen the muscles of the pelvic floor. Men achieve that relaxation and lengthening through the intrarectal massage only.

For either form of the internal massage, use a lubricant first; again, it should be paraben-free and without propylene glycol. Also, it may be easier and more comfortable to use a dilator. Whether you use your finger or the dilator, you will only penetrate from about half an inch to three inches deep. Again, as the pain subsides over time, increase the pressure gradually.

Intravaginal Internal Pelvic Floor Self-Massage for Women. Lie back comfortably with your knees bent, feet flat. Place pillows under both knees if that's more comfortable. Visualize the area you are probing as a clock. Your pubic bone is the 12 o'clock position, and the anus is at 6 o'clock. (It might help to use a mirror as you visualize the clock.) Insert your finger or the dilator to a depth of about an inch and start at the 6 o'clock position.

Now move gently and slowly counterclockwise to the 2 o'clock position, probing thoroughly for sore points. Then go the other way, clockwise, testing the area from 6 o'clock to 10 o'clock. As with the external massage, when you hit a sore point, apply pressure or knead it—very gently, as these muscles and tissues are highly sensitive—for at least 30 and at most 90 seconds. Then move on. You can go as far back into the vaginal canal as three inches to assess the different muscles of the pelvic floor, but be careful to be gentle with yourself.

You never want to probe the area between the 10 o'clock and 2 o'clock positions, directly below the pelvic bone. The reason? That's an organ—namely, the urethra and bladder—and should not be pressed. Leave this area for professionals to assess.

Otherwise, massaging your sore points is an essential part of the healing process. Be sure to do it every day.

The Intrarectal Internal Pelvic Floor Self-Massage for Men and Women. Lie back comfortably with your knees bent, feet flat—with or without pillows under your knees. For the intrarectal massage, the perineal body is at the 12 o'clock position and the tailbone or coccyx is at 6 o'clock. Insert your finger or the dilator to a depth of about an inch, and start at the 5 o'clock position. Move your finger or the dilator gently and slowly counterclockwise from 5 o'clock to 1 o'clock, probing thoroughly for sore points. Then go to the other side, testing the area clockwise from 7 o'clock to 11 o'clock. As with the external massage, when you hit a sore point, apply pressure or knead—very gently—for at least 30 and at most 90 seconds. Then move on. Here too, you can go as far back as three inches to assess the different muscles and tissues of the pelvic floor. Once you get comfortable with the "clock," you may find it more comfortable to lie on your side with your knees bent and a pillow or two between your knees.

Men should never probe the area between the 11 o'clock and 1 o'clock positions because that is the area where the prostate is—basically, at 12 o'clock. Neither gender should probe the area between 5 o'clock and 7 o'clock because that is the location of the tailbone, and massaging bone can be painful, although it is not harmful to do so. Again, leave these areas to the professionals.

THE ILU SELF-MASSAGE

Many of my patients refer to the ILU massage as the I Love You massage. The reason it's called ILU is that your massage movements will trace the shapes of those letters.

The ILU massage targets the colon—specifically the descending, transverse, and ascending colon, as shown in Figure 5.1. If your colon is blocked—if you have constipation, diarrhea, or irritable bowel syndrome or any similar discomfort—the ILU massage works like a charm. But you don't have to have any symptoms at all

Figure 5.1 Anatomy of the Colon for "ILU" Massage

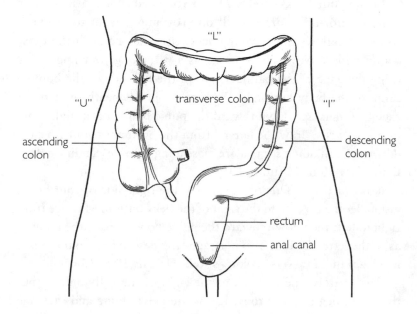

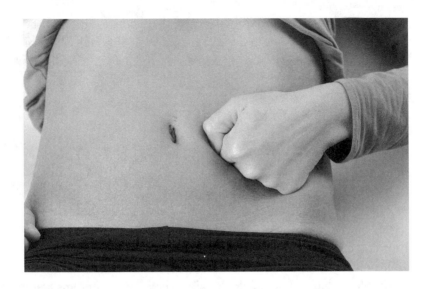

to benefit from the ILU massage. It's just an excellent way to relax your core and keep it healthy. Here's how to do it:

Lie on your back—preferably on your bed, but a firm sofa or other comfortable surface will do. You might want to wedge a couple of pillows under your knees. Use your hand in the most comfortable way possible—either as a fist, using your fingers, or using the edge of the palm. Begin on the left side of the body— think of the belly button as the center—just beneath the left rib cage, and massage down toward the pubic bone in a straight line. In other words, draw the letter *I* from the bottom of your rib cage downward. In doing so, you are massaging your descending colon. Draw the *I* 10 to 15 times.

Now for the *L*. This time, start on the right side of your body, just under the rib cage to the right of the belly button. Massage from right to left, then down toward the pubic bone: across, then down, as in the letter *L*. This also massages the descending colon, but it massages the transverse colon as well. Do this 10 to 15 times.

Finally, draw the *U*. Start to the right of the belly button, but this time, begin at the top edge of the pelvic bone and massage *up* toward the right side of the rib cage, then across to the left, then down to the top of the pelvic bone. Repeat 10 to 15 times. This adds the ascending colon to the massage. Thus, in drawing all three letters, you effectively massage your entire colon—descending, transverse, and ascending.

Use moderate pressure at most—lighter pressure if you have discomfort or diarrhea. Remember that you are not just stroking your skin; you are trying to get to the soft tissue beneath the skin. You need to feel this massage, but you don't want it to hurt. If you feel no pressure, you're probably not massaging hard enough. If you feel pain, you're massaging too hard, and you should lighten the pressure. Be aware that any kind of massage can produce soreness the next day, so by all means begin gently. And again: if you're feeling any pain at all, lighten up the pressure or stop the massage altogether.

I often suggest to my patients that they end the ILU massage with a post-massage that just circles the belly button and massages the small intestine. (Do this clockwise, which is the direction of the small intestine.) It also feels good.

So lie back, relax, pamper yourself. Let go. Your aim isn't to get this massage over with; your aim is to be good to yourself by caring for your body's core. Do it carefully and lovingly. It's all part of the healing.

CHAPTER 6

EAT RIGHT FOR A HEALTHY PELVIC FLOOR

It's not exactly headline news that diet affects health. Today, we're bombarded by advice about what to eat, when to eat, and how to eat to stay healthy. We're told by everybody from government guidelines writers to gourmet chefs to focus on plant foods, avoid saturated fats, stay away from sugars, limit processed foods, balance our protein and carbs, and eat in moderation. It's all excellent advice, and the fact is, what's good for our overall health, nutritionally speaking, is also good for pelvic floor health.

But it is also the case that some foods and some ways of eating are particularly helpful if you have a pelvic floor disorder, while some other foods and ways of eating can be particularly irritating to the disorder. To the extent that irritating a disorder can slow down your healing process, eating the right foods in the right way can be seen as an important way to support the healing you're doing with the exercise and massage programs you're undertaking. That's what this chapter is about. It offers guidelines for what to emphasize and what to avoid to make sure you get the most out of the natural healing process you've begun.

I'm going to assume that you know how to read a nutrition label—that you understand that serving size is the key to the label, for example, and that you know the basic nutritional definitions. I'm also going to assume that you have no known food allergies or, if you do, that you are under a doctor's care for the treatment of these allergies. And certainly, if you are suffering from a specific pelvic floor dysfunction, you should consult with your health-care practitioner about precisely what you should eat and what you should avoid eating to deal with your individual condition.

But if you're reading this book because you have a pelvic floor disorder that is causing you pain or problems, there are some general nutritional guidelines you can follow and some specific tips for bladder and bowel disorders. All of these guidelines are also general good-health recommendations; following them will help you to have a healthy pelvic floor and a healthy body for life.

GENERAL GUIDELINES FOR PELVIC FLOOR NUTRITION

Generally speaking, anything that makes digestion easier—anything that calms the gut—is good for you if you're experiencing pelvic floor disorder. Keep in mind, for example, that cooked foods are easier to digest than raw foods, while still offering sufficient nutrition. Something else that's very good for the digestion is to eat four to five smaller meals scattered throughout the day rather than three big meals morning, noon, and night. Both sides of the equation ease the digestive process: the fact that you are eating less at any one time, and the fact that you are allowing time for the smaller portions to be digested between meals.

What should you eat at those smaller, more frequent meals? The government-issued food pyramid sanctioned by the Department of Agriculture—http://www.mypyramid.gov—is a good place to start, with its recommendations for five servings of fruits and vegetables every day, four servings of whole grains, and moderate amounts of protein.

The fruits and veggies are particularly important if you have pelvic floor disorder because they add fiber to the diet, and fiber is key in advancing the digestive process. In fact, it's advisable to have some 20 to 35 grams of soluble and insoluble fiber daily to ensure the smooth running of your digestive tract. Twenty to 35 grams is really not that much in terms of weight; 35 grams is just a little over an ounce of food.

What are soluble and insoluble fiber? Soluble fiber disperses in water and slows down the process of digestion through the intestinal tract, whereas insoluble fiber—what we typically think of as "roughage"—doesn't break down easily and thus speeds the process.

Soluble fiber is found in cereals, fruits, and colorful vegetables like carrots and broccoli, beans, and peas.

Some Common Sources of Soluble Fiber

Cereal grains: barley, oatmeal, oat bran
Seeds: psyllium, flax
Fruit: pears, citrus fruits, apples, peaches, plums, and more
Beans: lima, black, navy, pinto, lentils
Peas: chickpeas, black-eyed peas
Vegetables: carrots, broccoli

For insoluble fiber, look for the leafy green vegetables, root vegetables, nuts, and whole wheat products—and be aware that if a product is truly whole wheat, the label will say so by putting "100% whole wheat" first in its listing. The skins of fruits and of root vegetables in particular are also excellent sources of insoluble fiber. One caution about insoluble fiber: if you have abdominal cramps, foods rich in insoluble fiber can exacerbate your pain, so eat them in moderation or stick to soluble fiber instead; it is easier to digest. Ditto if you have constipation or diarrhea: in either case, you can eat insoluble fiber, but you want to limit it initially. After your constipation or diarrhea calms down, then you can add more insoluble fiber—slowly and carefully.

Some Common Sources of Insoluble Fiber
Fruits: fruit skins, berries, grapes, prunes
Vegetables: beets, carrots, brussels sprouts, cabbage, cauliflower, broccoli
Other: kidney beans, bran

Some foods contain both soluble and insoluble fiber—broccoli, carrots, some fruits. The key is that foods containing insoluble fiber are harder to digest than those containing only soluble fiber. This means if you're having digestive problems, avoid foods containing insoluble fiber—at least at first until the digestive problem calms down.

But just as important as the foods that provide particular benefit to the health of your pelvic floor are the foods that can harm your healing. Specifically, try to avoid the simple carbohydrates or simple sugars. You know the foods I mean: cakes, candy, white bread, cookies, and the like. Also to be avoided are other "white" products—the starches like white flour, white rice, plain pasta, and white potatoes that can inject added yeast into your system. In addition, these foods can cause constipation, which of course is totally detrimental to digestion. There is also some speculation that too much of these sugars and starches can increase inflammation in the body and exacerbate the symptoms of such conditions as endometriosis. As for artificial sweeteners, unfortunately, they're no better, as they tend to irritate the gut and the bladder both.

It's also a good idea to limit your intake of alcohol and caffeine, both of which dehydrate the body, and both of which can aggravate bladder problems. Sometimes, it is true, an alcoholic drink can relax the muscles, including the pelvic floor muscles, and sometimes a cup of coffee or tea can help to stimulate a bowel movement and thus ease constipation. But as a general rule, both alcohol and caffeine are best in moderation—for any number of health reasons!—and there are, of course, other ways to relax the pelvic floor muscles and ease constipation.

Instead, drink plenty of nonalcoholic and noncaffeinated fluids. Six to eight glasses a day will keep the body hydrated. The taller and bigger you are, or the more you tend to perspire, the more you should drink. Moreover, if you have bladder or bowel issues, it's essential to take in plenty of these fluids.

Avoid fried foods and foods high in saturated fat whenever and wherever possible; that's good advice for health in general, but it's also true that these foods can contribute to clogged arteries, which decrease blood flow. If you have a pelvic floor disorder, chances are the blood flow to the pelvic region is already constricted because of pelvic congestion or tight muscles, so fried and fatty foods will only make the situation worse. What's more, you need good nutrition to help your healing process, and fried foods and foods high in saturated fats simply don't qualify as nutritional.

For those women who suffer vulvar vestibulitis, one more set of foods to think about avoiding is those high in oxalates. Oxalates occur naturally in certain foods such as blackberries, blueberries, raspberries, strawberries, spinach, Swiss chard, beet greens, collards, okra, almonds, cashews, peanuts, legumes, grains, even hot chocolate—many of the foods otherwise considered good for overall health and for pelvic floor health as well. Yet recent research suggests that the acid content of oxalates can increase the pain and skin irritation that can occur in the vestibule of the vagina in women. And while the verdict is still out on this claim, it's important to be aware of the possibility if this is a condition you experience.

If you are changing your diet to help heal pelvic floor disorders, be aware that it may take at least one month—and more probably, anywhere from three to six months—for you to notice a change in your bladder or bowel. If after eight months there is no significant change, or if you are not satisfied with your progress, you should consult with a nutritionist or with a health-care provider who specializes in nutrition as it affects bowel, bladder, and chronic pain issues.

IF YOU HAVE BLADDER PROBLEMS

If stress incontinence is your problem, follow these guidelines as best you can:

1. Drink at least six and preferably eight 8-ounce glasses of noncaffeinated, nonalcoholic beverages a day. Water is the top choice, but juices or herbal teas are also okay. But do try to finish your last intake of liquid at least two hours prior to bedtime.
2. Limit or eliminate caffeine and acidic teas like green tea. These act as diuretics or bladder irritants that can result in increased urinary frequency, and the acid can be just as irritating to the bladder as the caffeine in these drinks.
3. Avoid constipation. It results in increased pressure on the bladder. See the next section, "If You Have Bowel Problems," for more detail on how to avoid constipation.

If your problem is irritated or painful bladder or urge incontinence, do all of the above, and add the following food no-nos. While not everybody is affected by these foods in the same way, all of them have a tendency to aggravate the symptoms of irritation and urge incontinence, so to the extent possible, try to avoid the following:

- Acidic foods and beverages like most citrus fruits and fruit drinks as well as wines that contain tannins
- Spicy foods

- Carbonated beverages: the bubbles tend to aggravate the bladder
- Yeast-producing foods such as white bread, white rice, candy, or cake

Here's a way to counterbalance something you have eaten that you know may aggravate your bladder: put a quarter-teaspoon of baking soda into a big glass of water, and drink it down. Then drink another glass of water. The solution will help alkalinize your urine—that is, counter the acidity of what you've eaten. Be careful if you have any sort of heart condition or high blood pressure, however, as the baking soda has a high salt content. Instead, just make sure you avoid the aggravating food in the first place.

IF YOU HAVE BOWEL PROBLEMS

Constipation and diarrhea are the two main bowel problems that can be helped—or exacerbated—by what you eat. Both are certainly unpleasant and often painful, and both constitute burdens on the digestive process.

Constipation

Constipation can result in increased abdominal pressure, bloating, gas, and pressure on the bladder, the pelvic organs, and the pelvic floor muscles. Severe constipation results in increased toxicity in the bowel and in the body.

The straining that constipation gives rise to is particularly bad for you: it increases abdominal pressure, stresses the pelvic floor muscles, and could result in a hernia of the abdomen or pelvic floor muscles or pelvic organ prolapse. Here's a good way to picture it: if you have any problems with the pelvic floor muscles at all, and you strain because of constipation, it is like running a marathon with a bad knee. In other words, you could be causing real, long-term harm.

How do you get constipation? The main causes are insufficient fiber in the diet, insufficient liquids, insufficient exercise, too many simple sugars or white products, and certain diseases. Medications very often cause constipation, so be aware of this when your doctor writes you a prescription. Tight pelvic floor muscles may cause the bowel retention that can contribute to constipation.

In addition, some people have specific food intolerances that, when cured, lead to relief of bowel symptoms—an indication that these intolerances may cause the symptoms in the first place. Some folks may be gluten intolerant, unable to digest the substance found in most cereals and whole grains. Others may be lactose intolerant; in their case, the enzyme lactase, which breaks down the milk sugar lactose, is diminished or missing in the digestive tract, often leading to bloating and abdominal cramping. In both cases, curing the intolerance—or simply giving up the particular food—cures the bowel issue and ends the constipation. There are medical tests for both of these intolerances—or you can simply try doing without gluten and/or milk products for a time and seeing if your symptoms improve.

Nutritional Guidelines for Constipation. You will need to take nutritional steps to activate the gut in case of constipation. But don't make a radical change in your diet. That is, if you mostly eat high-fat foods and white foods, don't suddenly switch to a high-fiber diet; that will be a shock to the system that may actually exacerbate your symptoms. Ease into the changes instead:

1. Add fiber to your daily diet slowly, working your way incrementally to the recommended 35 grams per day. At first, focus on the soluble fiber contained in fruits, vegetables, and oatmeal rather than on the insoluble, which, although good for you, can make bowel movements harder and more difficult to pass. As your gut calms, slowly

begin to add insoluble fiber to your diet, and maintain a daily balance between soluble and insoluble fiber.

2. Eliminate fried foods and foods high in fat.
3. Drink plenty of water.
4. Eat the government-recommended five servings a day of fruits and vegetables along with moderate amounts of healthy protein, but avoid gas-producing foods like broccoli and dried fruits.
5. Limit simple carbs, starches, and artificial sweeteners.
6. Try probiotics—dietary supplements containing good bacteria that benefit digestion.

Gas-Producing Foods to Avoid If Constipated

Asparagus
Beans and other legumes: baked beans, chickpeas, kidney beans, lentils, lima beans, navy beans, pinto beans
Broccoli
Brussels sprouts
Cabbage
Cauliflower
Corn
Cucumbers
Dried fruits
Leeks
Peas
Peppers
Prunes
Carbonated drinks
Beer
Red wine
Fried and fatty foods
Sugar substitutes
Dairy products

Here's another important tip, although not a matter of nutrition: engage in some cardiovascular activity. It's muscle-enhancing exercise, and since muscle expends more energy and uses more calories than fat, the exercise helps to quicken the metabolism. That in turn speeds elimination and can calm the gut.

If all of these actions still don't solve the problem, add one of the many over-the-counter treatments for constipation. Typically, these contain psyllium (Metamucil), methylcellulose preparation (Citrucel), or a hydrating laxative (milk of magnesia). Use any of these treatments sparingly and temporarily; abuse can worsen your underlying problem.

Diarrhea

Diarrhea can be dehydrating and, if it lasts for any period of time, downright dangerous. The trick to avoiding it or healing it is to find the happy medium between too much fiber, which can cause diarrhea, and not enough fiber causing constipation. Since everyone's body is different and responds differently to various food products, finding that happy medium isn't always easy.

Once it's found, however, the nutritional guidelines for diarrhea are much the same as those for constipation; all are aimed at calming the gut.

Nutritional Guidelines for Diarrhea. Here are some simple steps you can take to combat diarrhea.

1. Start by reducing the amount of fiber in your diet in order to get the diarrhea under control. Then, reintroduce soluble fiber slowly into your diet to avoid constipation. Once you're able to tolerate the soluble fiber, slowly add small portions of insoluble fiber until you work up to a balance

between the two. If you cannot tolerate insoluble fiber at all, stick to the soluble fiber.

2. Eliminate fried foods and those with high fat content.
3. Drink plenty of water.
4. Limit sugars, starches, and artificial sweeteners.
5. Try for the government recommendation of five servings of fruits and vegetables per day along with healthy protein.
6. Try probiotics.

Again, if these guidelines don't work, try an over-the-counter antidiarrhea medication. Start with a small amount; too big a dose can lead to constipation.

YOUR FOOD DIARY

One of the best ways to understand how to keep your digestion calm—and your pelvic floor in good working order—is to keep a food diary.

The key to a successful food diary is to be completely conscientious about filling it out: every meal, every drink, every snack. Only in that way can you begin to see connections between what you eat and any discomfort or disorder. Also, it takes time. Patterns don't emerge overnight.

In the following food diary, you can keep track of everything you eat, noting what you eat and what time you eat it, and everything you drink and when you drink it. You should also note any discomfort you feel or disorder that occurs: again, what it is and when you first felt it.

Be patient and persistent in monitoring your intake and any consequences. In due course, your food diary will show you what aggravates your digestive tract and what soothes it—and you'll be better equipped to ensure a healthy pelvic floor.

	Food	Time	Drink	Time	Discomfort/ Disorder	Time
Sunday						
Monday						
Tuesday						
Wednesday						
Thursday						
Friday						
Saturday						

ADDITIONAL RESOURCES

There is lots more information available on specific foods that can harm or potentially heal specific conditions. Moreover, the research on these issues is ongoing—and at a pretty fast pace. That's why it's important to check with your health-care provider about any specific condition you know you have to discuss which foods to avoid and which to emphasize.

I also recommend checking online with the association that addresses your particular condition. These associations—for example, the National Vulvodynia Association (www.nva.org), the Interstitial Cystitis Association (www.ichelp.com), the Irritable Bowel Syndrome Association (www.ibsassociation.org), and many others (see Appendix B)—tend to be current on the very latest research and can potentially offer the most up-to-date nutritional recommendations.

In general, however, it's important to keep in mind that a healthy, low-fat diet, one that limits simple carbs and is rich in fiber and other basic nutrients, can keep your pelvic floor healthy. And a healthy pelvic floor is the core of a healthy you.

CHAPTER 7

RELAX AND TAKE CARE OF YOURSELF

Stress and pelvic floor disorders turn together in a vicious circle. Relaxing and taking care of yourself are therefore a critical part of the natural way to healing.

As we have seen, tension and anxiety, whether from a traumatic event or from the strains and worries that are scattered through every life, tend to "settle" in the core of the body, shortening and tightening the muscles of the pelvic floor, the back, and the abdomen and leading to the cascade of pain and dysfunction we've talked about earlier.

Such stress also sets up a physiological response that can suppress the immune system. When that happens, any area of the body that is already weak or in pain becomes something of a target—that is, it's more susceptible than ever to infection, to further weakening, to more tension, to other problems.

Moreover, stress can keep you from sleeping well, and since sleep is the time when your body repairs itself and renews its tissues, the stress of pelvic floor disorders can work against the healing process. In fact, insomnia contributes significantly to the suppression of the immune system as well.

The bottom line is that stress is particularly bad for you if you have a pelvic floor dysfunction or weak pelvic floor muscles. It usually makes the condition worse, and it contributes to the rotating cascade of pain the dysfunction or weakness gives rise to. So for any diagnosis of pelvic disorder, pain, or weakness, learning how to manage your stress and practicing self-care to stay relaxed are essential prescriptions.

But managing stress can mean all sorts of different things to different people, and it's important to keep in mind not just that everybody is different, but that every *body* is different. We all have our own DNA signature, as individual to us as our fingerprints, and we all respond in different ways to stress and the processes for reducing stress. I know lots of people who swear by meditation. I know others who need a hot bath and soothing music. Some people chill out by watching a funny movie, while others head to the gym for a sweaty workout. For me, it takes some stretching and deep breathing or some form of cardiovascular exercise like Rollerblading, snowboarding, or skiing to clear my head, reinvigorate my energy level, and get rid of the strains and anxieties that come with running a business, managing a household, caring for patients, and being engaged in personal relationships with family and friends.

The point is that whatever works to relax you and lower your stress will also help heal your pelvic floor disorder—and, most of the time, vice versa. (Of course, all the exercises of the End-the-Pain and Strengthen-the-Muscles routines you learned in Chapters 3 and 4 and the massage therapies of Chapter 5 are key to managing stress and healing pelvic floor disorders.) Still, this chapter will focus on methods that have proven particularly effective in lengthening and relaxing the pelvic floor, surrounding muscles, and the nervous system to send the tension and pain packing. So regard the suggestions in this chapter as just that—suggestions. None of them can do you any harm whatsoever; all have the potential to do you good. The important thing is to see what works for you and then to make those techniques and self-care initiatives a part of your healing program—and a part of your life.

FIRST, BREATHE

Actually, back in Chapter 3, you already learned what is perhaps the most important—and certainly the most basic—stress management technique there is: deep breathing. Here's a refresher course:

- *Inhale.* Expand your belly outward and your ribs to the sides and "open" your pelvic floor, without lifting your chest. Feel the air filling the "receiving area" of your lungs, making one big chamber. Inhale for three to five seconds.
- *Exhale.* Start from the top. Let the air out of your upper lungs, then relax your ribs, your belly, and your pelvic floor so that the air just gradually flows out of you. Exhale for four to six seconds.

I've already recommended that you start every day with deep breathing and that you make it a key part of your exercise program. In addition, do it whenever you feel particularly tense, when you note that your breathing has grown shallow and quick, or when you feel anxious in your mind or body.

Deep breathing requires no special tools. You can do it anywhere and at any time. And it's absolutely free. Yet it's one of the most effective ways I know of to calm your nerves, banish anxiety from your body and mind, and relieve pain and muscle tension. Whenever you feel stressed, your first move should be to take a deep breath.

TIPS FOR THE TOILET

If you suffer from any of the bladder or bowel problems listed in Chapter 3—urgency, frequency, retention, or pain—here are some tips for relaxing when you are on the toilet.

To begin with, one good way to relax the pelvic floor is to place a stool underneath your feet as you are seated on the toilet. Use a couple of phone books if you don't have a stool the right height.

Then, don't rush it, and don't strain. Breathe, and try to relax.

Instead, if your issue is your bladder, try massaging the area right over the bladder—the lower center of the abdomen just above the pubic bone. Use any of the techniques you learned in Chapter 5 and just stroke the area for a minute or so. If the bowel is your problem, do the ILU massage from Chapter 5—again, for a minute or so.

Relaxing in these ways can facilitate a more efficient emptying of your bladder and bowel.

THE KEY-IN-THE-LOCK SYNDROME: CONTROL THE URGE

Deep breathing can even help relieve bladder and bowel urgency and frequency as well as urge incontinence. Use it for what is called the key-in-the-lock syndrome. I'll explain:

If you drink a mug or two of coffee in the morning, the normal tendency is to feel the urge to urinate after about an hour. So if you feel the urge to urinate within 10 minutes of your cup of coffee, and then another 10 minutes after that, and again 10 minutes later, that is not normal.

It's just like what happens when you feel the urge to urinate, arrive home, and just as you are putting the key in the lock, you get an intense urge and you begin to leak—or to feel you are leaking, even if it is not the case.

What's going on—and how can you control these untimely and inconvenient urges?

Although it is called key-in-the-lock, the real name for this is urgency-frequency syndrome or urge incontinence—the feeling that you have to go and that you will not be able to hold it in till you reach a toilet. It is both a cause and a result of stress; in fact, it's one of the most stressful things an individual confronts, with the worry about its future occurrence as bad as the urge itself. What can you do about it?

First, as noted, deep-breathe and drop the pelvic floor muscles five to 10 times. Although it seems counterintuitive to relax the muscles when you feel a strong urge, it works. If your pelvic floor muscles are already shortened, and you are tightening them every time you have the urge, then you are shortening the muscles even more and are fatiguing them as well, which is precisely what can lead to urgency-frequency syndrome and/or urge incontinence.

Second, think thoughts that can relax you. One good bet is to visualize a place where you have felt utterly relaxed and at ease. Maybe it's that tropical beach where you vacationed a couple of years ago. Maybe it's a cabin in the North Woods where you've always hoped to get snowed in. Picture the place—palm trees and white sand, or deep snowdrifts and a warm fire. In your mind, place yourself there. Now relax.

In the beginning, you are only trying to control the urge for a brief time—another 10 minutes perhaps. You are not trying to "hold it in" for the full hour considered "normal" after drinking coffee, or for an exaggerated distance to the nearest bathroom. Ten more minutes this week, maybe another 10 next week as the muscles learn to relax through practice, then another five the week after—and so on. In due course, you will have taught your muscles to relax and lengthen so that the urgency will abate.

As you retrain your pelvic floor muscles, be sure to take care of the rest of your body as well, for doing so enhances the healing of your pelvic floor. The best place to practice total-body stress reduction and self-care is in the privacy and comfort of your own home.

YOUR HOME SPA AND OTHER STRESS-REDUCTION TECHNIQUES

You can pay a fortune to go to an upscale destination resort spa—or you can practice stress reduction for free, in your own neighborhood and right in your own home.

You might start off your relaxing time with a walk in the park—maybe just a languid stroll today, or maybe a brisk constitutional to get your circulation going. Both can reduce stress.

Top it off when you get home with a hot bath. Fill the tub, light the candles, turn on the music, turn off the telephone, and sink down into the water. Let the heat suffuse your body till you can feel yourself relaxing. Empty your mind. Listen only to the music, not to that to-do list in your head. This is your time; take advantage of it. When you're ready to climb out, stretch the warmth with a cup of tea—maybe chamomile or mint, which calm the stomach—to relax you even further. Dress in loose-fitting clothing; tight clothing can increase skin irritations and can decrease blood flow. Sit down in your favorite chair. Special cushions to alleviate pain in your tailbone, sit-bone area, or perineum may help; search on "sitting cushions" on the Internet for sources. Read a book. Write a letter. Watch a movie.

Maybe yoga is your thing: loose clothing, a mat on the floor, quiet time to focus on the postures.

Do you know how to do meditation? It isn't hard to learn, but there is a right way to do it—and many books, tapes, and online courses that teach the right way. Once you learn how, it's a great way to gain a sense of calm and stability that lasts. And, like deep breathing, it's something you can do anywhere, any time for a few minutes to get a quick hit of stress reduction.

TECHNIQUES FOR SOOTHING THE PELVIC FLOOR

Interested in some special techniques for soothing the pelvic area? Try lying down on your back and elevating your pelvis with pillows or a wedge. Especially if you have the kind of job that keeps you on your feet all day, this can help improve your circulation and reverse the blood flow away from your pelvic area where it has probably congested during the day.

While you're lying there, give yourself what's called an effleurage massage. Put some oil or lotion on your fingertips or palms and just gently stroke your abdomen and pelvic region. This massage warms and relaxes the muscles and helps to improve blood flow.

For even more relaxing warmth, use a hot water bottle or heating pad. Place the bottle or pad right on the abdomen to help relax your bladder and bowel. Or, lying on your stomach, place the bottle or pad on the tailbone or back right on top of any pelvic pain you may be suffering to loosen muscle tightness, increase blood flow, and relax the muscles. If you suffer from any sort of bladder urgency, frequency, or pain, or if you're experiencing constipation, diarrhea, or irritable bowel, applying heat in this way can calm the gut and relax the muscles as well. You can do this warmth therapy as often as you like and throughout the day, but do not place a heating pad on your belly if you are pregnant or if you have any condition for which the application of heat is contraindicated.

If your skin is irritated anywhere around the anal region, or if you're a woman who has pain at penetration during sex, or if you suffer from tailbone or any pelvic pain, try a contrast bath: stroke the affected area with an ice cube for one minute—be sure to move it around so it doesn't burn your skin, then apply a warm washcloth for one minute. The ice cools and thus decreases the inflammation and calms muscle spasm, while the warmth increases the blood flow and relaxes tight muscles and tissues. So both assist the healing process. That is why you should repeat the procedure anywhere from three to five times, and do it up to three times a day.

Any and all of these methodologies can help heal your pelvic floor disorder because they help relax the mind and banish tension from the body. They cost little or no money; they don't require the involvement of others; they don't call for any special equipment. No doubt there are other things you like to do to relax. Whichever techniques work for you, incorporate them into your life; they're an important part of healing your pelvic floor disorder, and they're important for your overall health as well.

ONGOING CARE: POSTURE AND ALIGNMENT

One of the best ways to take care of yourself to ensure a healthy pelvic floor for life is to maintain proper posture and body alignment. The reason is simple: poor posture and muscle imbalance can cause and certainly contribute to pelvic floor dysfunction. Think about it: if your body is not properly aligned, if you slouch or are off balance, your organs are off balance and out of alignment as well. Your muscles are shortened where they should be long and are lengthened where they should be short, and the bottom line is that your body is simply not functioning effectively or efficiently. Here's why:

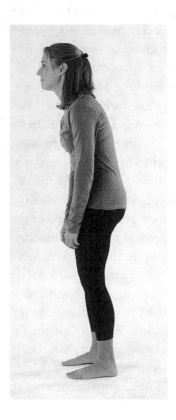
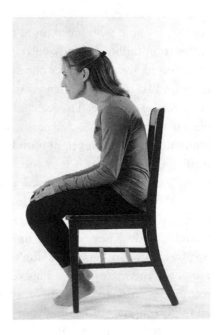

Our joints contain nerve endings called proprioceptors that tell us where we are in space. If you have spent years slouching, for example, with your head forward and your shoulders rounded, your body's proprioception may now accept the slouching as the norm. In this norm, however, your abdominal muscles have shortened and reduced the space in your abdominal cavity where your pelvic organs reside; the result is there's less mobility in the abdominal cavity. Your slouched norm has also resulted in lengthening your back muscles, which now have a difficult time contracting efficiently. Your posture is forcing your back muscles to work harder, and chances are good you have fairly chronic back pain.

That proprioception is going to be hard to break through after all these years, so you'll need to do posture exercises frequently and on a regular basis till you retrain your nerve endings and reeducate your muscles to good posture and proper alignment. Do the following exercises three times daily at first, then once a day for your lifetime. All you need is a wall.

1. Stand against the wall with your shoulders back so that your shoulder blades, head, buttocks, and heels are all touching the wall. Look straight ahead. Bend your knees slightly, and contract your abdominal muscles very gently; do not suck in your stomach, just bring your belly button toward your spine. This is the easy part of the exercise. Now, hold the posture, and try to memorize what it feels like in your body. (If you have a full-length mirror, it can be helpful to position it so that by turning your head, you can see the side view of yourself holding the posture.) Got it? Okay, now take a couple steps away from the wall. Try to maintain the posture as you do so, and try to maintain it throughout the day, but be careful not to hold yourself too stiff. Maintaining the posture without the help of the wall is the hard part of the exercise. You will probably need to remind yourself of how the posture felt in your body multiple times until it becomes a habit, as it will in time.

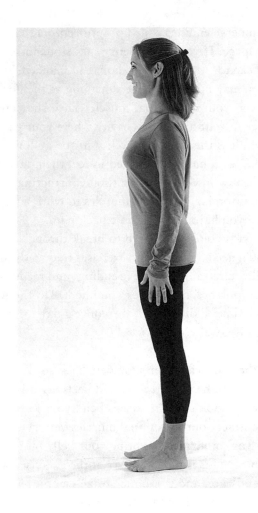

2. Do the same thing seated. (If you have any pain, try sitting on a cushion or a pillow.) Sit against a wall with your shoulder blades, head, and buttocks touching the wall. Look straight ahead. Gently contract your abdomen by bringing your belly button toward your spine—do not suck in your stomach. Memorize how the posture feels, and try to maintain it while sitting at your desk or commuting by bus or train or in whatever sitting you do during the day. A lumbar cushion may help, as is shown in the photo.

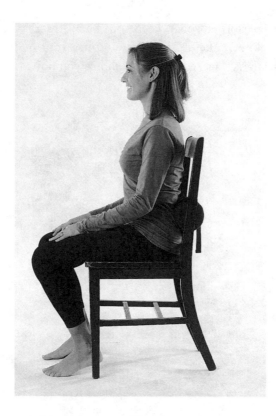

At first as you do these exercises, you may find that you need to remind yourself of what the posture feels like repeatedly during the course of a day. You may also find that you can only hold the posture, standing or seated, for a few minutes or even a few seconds at a time. But I promise you that as you keep at it, you will improve. Next week, you'll only need to remind yourself of the posture 10 times a day, and you may be able to maintain the posture for 10 minutes at a stretch. Remember: it is a matter of reeducating your muscles out of bad habits and retraining your body's proprioceptors. It takes time—and practice.

In addition to standing properly, it's important to lift properly. The following photo demonstrates poor lifting. Lift from the legs; don't use your back. Stand as close as possible to the item to be lifted. Then perform a squat: keep your back straight, bend at the hip and the knee, take up the item, and use your abdominals to stand up straight. The second photo shows you how.

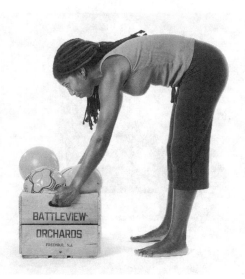

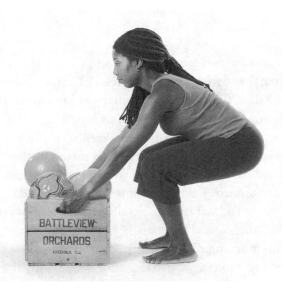

GETTING SUPPORT

An important part of the self-care that can keep you healthy at the core is emotional support. As has been noted, the whole topic of pelvic floor disorders has been "hush-hush" for years, and you can't get the support you need if you can't talk about the problem. In fact, one of the reasons I've written this book is in hopes of making pelvic floor pain and disorder an accepted topic of conversation, for only in that way can people who suffer the disorders find the healing they need.

The first place to go for support is to family members or friends. Not only will they be understanding; you are also likely to learn that someone you know is also suffering from some form of pelvic floor dysfunction or has suffered from it in the past. These are your nearest and dearest; they love you and don't want you to be in pain and discomfort, or to feel embarrassed or ashamed. Talk to them.

But family and friends are not your only resource. In fact, while family and friends will offer the support of love and comfort, you may need more direct professional guidance to deal with the impact of your dysfunction on your life. And if you are someone who simply is not comfortable talking to a friend or family member about your condition, a professional should be your first stop. Try to find a psychologist, social worker, psychiatrist, or other therapist who is familiar with pelvic pain and with urinary, bowel, or sexual dysfunction. If that particular expertise is not available where you live, then look for someone with specialized training in chronic pain or, at a minimum, in stress management. In addition, most studies show that cognitive behavioral therapy is an excellent technique for managing the stress and anxiety of pelvic floor disorder, so you might want to narrow your search to experts in that discipline. Many of the associations listed in Appendix B in the back of this book can help you find the right professional resource to meet your needs.

CHAPTER 8

BETTER SEX FOR MORE YEARS

Everybody wants a better sex life—and there's no shortage of advice on how to get one.

Some say it's a matter of position. Others say it's all about what you eat. Still others insist it's a question of hormones, pure and simple. There are those who tell you environment is everything and that at the right time of day, with the right mood music and appropriately scented candles, you can't miss. And of course, in this day and age, one of the most common prescriptions for better sex is to take a pill.

None of these suggestions is necessarily wrong. Yet one of the best ways to have a better sex life is also one of the simplest: strengthen your pelvic floor if it is weak, or stretch and relax it if the muscles have shortened or are tight.

The reason for the strengthening is simple: the muscles, nerves, and tissues that make up the pelvic floor are essential to sexual arousal and sexual fulfillment in both men and women. So it follows that the stronger and healthier your pelvic floor, the better your sexual performance and the more intense your sexual pleasure. In fact, just by doing the exercise program in Chapter 4 of this book, you're likely to improve your sexual skills and enhance your ability to enjoy the sexual experience.

Similarly, if your pelvic floor muscles have spasmed or short-ened, you may be feeling pain during or after intercourse. By fol-lowing the exercises in Chapter 3 of this book, and by doing the self-massage you learned in Chapter 5, you will be helping yourself to enjoy sex again.

In doing so, you'll do something else as well. By making your pelvic floor strong and supple—and by keeping it that way—you'll extend your sexual longevity. You won't just be enjoying sex more, you'll also be enjoying it for more years to come. And that will help you stay healthy for more years to come as well.

SEX, HEALTH, AND THE PELVIC FLOOR

There's a simple formula at work here: sex is important for good health, and health is important for good sex. Good sex and good health nurture and reinforce one another. And a healthy pelvic floor is key to both.

Why is sex good for us? Sexual activity increases the blood flow. That, in turn, equips the body to fight off such harmful bacterial infections and viruses as urinary tract and yeast infections, or to rid itself of them if they take hold. That helps keep our organs strong.

Sexual activity also helps our muscles stay strong. Orgasms, after all, are muscle contractions, so the more intense the orgasm, the greater the strengthening of the muscles. (And vice versa, of course: the stronger your pelvic floor muscles, the more intense your orgasm can be.) Strengthened muscles, in turn, mean lowered risk of incontinence. Orgasm also relaxes the body. And the stron-ger and less tense the muscles at our core, the less hard our bodies have to work to hold us upright.

Just as important as these physiological benefits are the psycho-logical and emotional payoffs of healthy sexual experiences. Sex, after all, is an essential component—some would say the crowning characteristic—of the kind of intimacy that is such a keystone of psychological and emotional well-being. It embodies and exemplifies that closeness to another that answers the most profound human need.

In so many ways, therefore, sex is very, very good for us, and that means that better sex is even better for us.

That's where the pelvic floor comes in. It is, after all, at the core of the body and as such, the seat of sex. The nerve endings of the pelvic floor are what respond to sexual stimulation. Its tissues and blood flow are where arousal takes place. Its muscles are literally the vehicles of sexual pleasure. In men, sexual arousal increases the sensitivity of the nerves and causes the tissues of the penis to become engorged with blood and thus erect. During orgasm, the male's pelvic muscles contract rapidly and rhythmically. In women, the main areas of sexual stimulation are the clitoris and the G-spot, the small area of tissue on the back wall of the vagina named for the German gynecologist Ernst Gräfenberg, who did groundbreaking research into female sexual physiology. The nerve endings of the pelvic floor muscles assist in the stimulation of these areas; they're the receptors of sexual excitement and arousal. Once a woman has become sexually aroused, the clitoris and G-spot engorge with blood, the nerve endings become more sensitive, and in turn the muscles of the pelvic floor contract.

But the specific muscle of the pelvic floor that is key to sexual pleasure in both men and women is the pubococcygeus, or PC muscle, which contracts rapidly during orgasm. So while a number of factors like hormone levels and positioning and the mood of the moment certainly affect sexual activity, the pelvic floor is clearly key to both performance and pleasure. A healthy pelvic floor—one with well-toned, relaxed muscles capable of going through their full range of motion, with a healthy blood flow nourishing healthy tissue, with nerve cells that respond well to stimulation—has all the ingredients necessary to ensure sensitivity to stimulation, powerful arousal, and highly satisfying climax. Bottom line: a healthy pelvic floor contributes to healthy sex, and healthy sex contributes to a healthy life.

SEXUAL DYSFUNCTION AND THE PELVIC FLOOR

Problems, dysfunctions, or weaknesses of the pelvic floor can adversely affect sexual performance and detract from sexual pleasure—and in turn from overall health and well-being in both men and women. If the pelvic floor's blood flow is insufficient, for example, the engorgement of the key areas of stimulation will also be insufficient, or may not take place. If the PC muscle is weak or if it has been shortened by tension—or both—it may respond only weakly during orgasm, if at all; it simply won't be able to go through the full range of motion that achieves a healthy and satisfying orgasm.

In some cases, these dysfunctions may be painful as well, and they can often undermine an individual's quality of life in disruptive, debilitating, and distressing ways. In men, erectile dysfunction (ED) and premature ejaculation are perhaps the best-known sexual dysfunctions. These days, you can't watch the nightly news or the weekly football game on television without being bombarded with ads for drugs that can remedy ED. In those cases where the disorder may result from decreased blood flow or from spasmed or weak muscles, a stronger, healthier pelvic floor may resolve the problem. Prostatitis—an inflammation of the prostate gland that can also decrease libido and cause impotence—is another fairly common male disorder, and it's been shown conclusively that 95 percent of its symptoms are nonbacterial and most likely caused by pelvic floor dysfunction.

It has also been shown conclusively that pelvic pain in men is also typically associated with sexual dysfunction. Studies have shown that more than 90 percent of men who suffer pelvic pain also experience sexual dysfunction, and that more than half of them improved their sexual function through massage of the pelvic floor muscles and relaxation techniques.

Women can suffer a range of sexual dysfunctions that are in great measure preventable if a healthy pelvic floor is maintained.

Traditionally, these dysfunctions were classified under the catch-all name *dyspareunia*, meaning pain that interferes with sexual activity. We now know that such pain is typically associated with some very specific disorders like vestibulitis, a skin irritation or inflammation at the opening or vestibule of the vagina that renders the area painful when touched; vulvodynia, a burning or stinging sensation felt throughout the vulva; or vaginismus, an involuntary spasm of some or all of the vaginal muscles. These painful conditions can turn sex into a painful experience for a woman; in fact, they can make it simply impossible.

Other sexual dysfunctions may affect both men and women: pain during and after sexual activity, decreased libido, and difficulty becoming stimulated and/or achieving orgasm. Clearly, these dysfunctions also affect the frequency of sexual activity, and they certainly affect the quality of life of both the affected individual and his or her partner.

Sometimes, these dysfunctions may be medically induced. Antidepressants, for example, as well as some pain medications and some cholesterol-lowering drugs, are known to decrease libido or otherwise diminish sexual activity and enjoyment. Similarly, stress and emotional challenges may reduce both the desire and the ability to have sex. The same goes for hormonal imbalance, which can lower sex drive and sexual ability in both men and women.

TAKING ACTION FOR A BETTER SEX LIFE

If you have any of the symptoms of these disorders, you should consult your physician immediately for a proper diagnosis. Like so many disorders, these may have their origin in pelvic floor dysfunctions that can be addressed by doing the natural healing methods in this book, but it's important to be sure. That isn't just sound medical practice; it's common sense. Doing exercises you should not do, or doing some exercises the wrong way, could actually add to or worsen your problems.

But for patients who receive their doctor's go-ahead, and certainly for people without symptoms of disorder or dysfunction, the exercises in this book offer not just a preventive hedge against future problems, but also a great way to enhance your sexual experience right now—and for years to come. If your problem is pain during or after intercourse, go to Chapter 3 and follow the End-the-Pain exercise routine, and do the self-massage therapies of Chapter 5. If your problem is difficulty achieving orgasm or decreased libido due to weak pelvic floor muscles—or if you want to intensify your sexual experience—follow the program of Chapter 4. Both programs will help you get healthy at the core, and as we've shown earlier, being healthy at the core is good for everything—good for your health in general and particularly good for your sex life.

There are some special things women can do to relieve vaginal irritation and pain. For those suffering irritation, for example, it can even be painful to wipe after urinating, and the solution is—don't. Instead, pat the skin, as you would a newborn baby's delicate skin; wiping is too aggressive on these sensitive tissues. Use scent-free babywash or, even better, plain water to wash the area. Gently. If you use a tampon, plastic applicators, with their smooth surface, are the better choice. If you're a swimmer irritated by the chlorine in the pool, apply Vaseline before you put on your bathing suit to protect this sensitive tissue. And try applying pure vitamin E oil twice a day for at least two months; this may ease the pain.

For women who experience pain during sex, positioning may ease the pain. While every individual's anatomy is different, the woman lying on her side with the man behind her is typically a less painful position for a woman who has experienced pain during intercourse. Some women also find that being on top is helpful since they can then control the angle of their posture and the speed of the action.

In any event, women who have had pain issues during sex should always use a lubricant, even once the pain begins to subside. There is a great variety of these products, so experiment to find the one that suits you best, but avoid any lube that contains propylene glycol, which tends to burn, and be sure that the lube you choose is paraben-free. Parabens are used as preservatives in many cosmetic and personal hygiene products and have been shown to mimic estrogen; they therefore may possibly contribute to the growth of tumors in the breast.

Women may also suffer incontinence during sex—and particularly at the point of orgasm, although of course it is important to differentiate female ejaculatory fluid from urinary incontinence. Urinary tract infections, yeast infections, or symptoms that mimic these infections are all common disorders that may result from sexual activity and, obviously, will interfere with sexual activity as well. It is important to get an accurate diagnosis: is it a urinary tract infection or a pelvic floor dysfunction? Is it a yeast infection or pelvic floor dysfunction? Don't self-diagnose; see your physician.

STRENGTHENING OR STRETCHING THE PELVIC FLOOR FOR BETTER SEX

The key to strengthening the pelvic floor is the Strengthen-the-Muscles exercises of Chapter 4—and most particularly, the Kegel. Indeed, while I've recommended Kegels as a way to avoid or cure incontinence, the fact is that Dr. Kegel was looking for a therapy to help women with sexual dysfunction when he came up with these exercises. Simply put, what Kegel found was that the more developed the vaginal muscles—specifically, the PC muscle—the more gratifying the sexual experience. The famous resistive exercise he devised develops the PC and the other pelvic floor muscles, increasing their contractile strength through voluntary control of their movement. And sure enough: as the PC muscle is developed through the Kegel exercises, becoming broader and thicker, the tone of the pelvic floor walls also increases, and the muscle's ability to contract in sexual response is substantively augmented.

Later research has repeatedly confirmed the validity of these conclusions. In fact, more recent studies that have sought to measure the difference in function between the undeveloped and developed PC muscle have yielded the dramatic finding that women with strong pelvic floor muscles enjoyed contractions two to three times more powerful than women with undeveloped muscles.

Kegel exercises also work for men. The voluntary contraction of the PC in the male engages what is called the cremasteric reflex; this lifts the testes and is a step in the sexual response cycle. Kegels may also enable multiple orgasms and can help prevent premature ejaculation.

But perhaps your problem isn't weakness but rather tightness, in which case you need to relax the muscles and free them of tension and of pain. That's where the exercises of Chapter 3 come in, as well as the self-massage techniques of Chapter 5. Lengthening the muscles and tissues of your pelvic floor and the surrounding area, reducing the points of irritation in the muscles, ridding the tissue of the toxins that cause even further tension, and increasing the flow of blood to the area all enhance your ability to become aroused and to enjoy the experience of sex.

The medical evidence is therefore undeniable: in both women and men, when the muscles and nerves of the pelvic floor are weak or dysfunctional, sexual response and sexual satisfaction are diminished. When the function of the muscles and nerves is improved through strengthening in the case of weakness, or through lengthening and massage in the case of pain and tension, both the interest in sexual activity and the satisfaction deriving from the activity rises dramatically.

For women in particular, we know today that a variety of orgasmic experiences is available to them along all those nerve pathways to the clitoris and the G-spot and in the muscle responses that can ensue. Following where the medical evidence leads, it's now clear that the program of exercise and other therapies in this book can enliven those pathways and enhance those muscle responses. Such a program can be the healthiest path possible to a much, much better sex life.

CHAPTER 9

PREGNANCY, LABOR, AND POSTDELIVERY

Pregnancy and labor put the pelvic floor muscles to the test. Don't worry—women with a history of pelvic floor disorders can still have a healthy, normal pregnancy and a quick return to their pre-pregnancy condition. For these nine months, your focus is quite naturally on your pelvis; that's where so many of the changes you're undergoing occur, and it's where a lot of your discomfort may originate. During pregnancy, your pelvic area has to continue to make room for the fetus growing inside you. Your body increases its production of the hormones relaxin and estrogen, which loosen the ligaments in the body and allow the pelvic bones to expand to accommodate the growing fetus. As a result, your joints are more lax. Also, your center of gravity shifts forward and your abdominal muscles lengthen—and in so doing lose some strength. Your back muscles, leg muscles, and pelvic floor muscles all have to work overtime to balance out the extra weight you're carrying and the change in your posture; this can cause neck pain, pelvic pain, back pain, and pain in the wrist, shoulder, and ankle.

As if all this weren't enough, your bladder is feeling the pressure of all these changes and of the growing fetus. You feel the urge to urinate more often, and many women experience some leaking.

Even though you probably won't experience all these bodily changes, any of them can be uncomfortable and disruptive. They can cause complications. Sometimes they're painful.

But of course, they're as normal and as natural as childbirth itself. And as you'll learn in this chapter, there is a lot you can do to mitigate the discomfort and to prepare your body for as smooth and easy a delivery and as rapid a return to prepregnancy normalcy as possible.

Keep this in mind: *You do not have to suffer.* You and your obstetrician will together work out what is best for you throughout the course of your pregnancy. But don't accept a "prescription" that tells you your pain will end "when the baby is born," especially if you're in the early stages of pregnancy. For one thing, that still leaves you plenty of time to be miserable; for another thing, the pain may not go away once the baby is born.

There is a lot you can do to help yourself. The relaxation techniques and exercises you've learned in this book—the same techniques and exercises that helped give you a healthy pelvic floor even before pregnancy—can also help alleviate your discomfort, keep you fit during pregnancy, provide you your best shot at a smooth, easy delivery, and help you get back into fighting trim after delivery as well. The exercises in this chapter are geared specifically to do all of that, and if you find that they are too easy, or if they become too easy as you continue to do them, you can give yourself more of a challenge by referring back to the appropriate section of Chapter 3, "Keeping the Exercises Challenging."

Such exercises may even help you conceive. Recent research has suggested that two possible causes of infertility may be related to the pelvic floor.

One possibility is pelvic congestion—that is, an insufficient or inadequate or ineffective flow of blood to the pelvic area and the pelvic organs. The congestion, in turn, could be the result of chronic inflammation or spasmed, overly tight muscles and tissues in the pelvis, abdomen, legs, and back.

A second possibility is a mechanical problem. Specifically, in those patients who experience pelvic pain, pelvic floor dysfunction, vestibulitis, and/or erectile dysfunction, there could be a correlation to spasmed muscles and an irritated nerve supply or adhesions that render intercourse difficult or even impossible.

Both of these possibilities are still very much in the research stage. But if infertility is an issue, it is worth discussing these issues with your health-care provider. In addition, I recommend seeking a full evaluation by a physical therapist who specializes in the treatment of pelvic floor dysfunction.

In any event, of course, you should discuss all of these techniques and exercises with your obstetrician; chances are he or she will applaud your initiative, but it's essential that you share what you are planning. And of course, pregnancy can produce or make you vulnerable to serious problems. For any muscle or bone pain or discomfort out of the ordinary, don't hesitate to see your physician or a physical therapist who specializes in pregnancy.

STAY FLEXIBLE AND STRONG

The natural way to stay fit during pregnancy, ease any discomfort you feel, smooth the delivery, and get you back to your prepregnancy state fast is really just a variation of the relaxation techniques and exercises you've learned elsewhere in this book. That's because staying both flexible and strong is key to keeping your pelvic floor healthy and fit, and a healthy and fit pelvic floor is the perfect preparation for what you're about to undergo in pregnancy and childbirth.

To begin with, it is important to stay flexible at all times, but perhaps never more so than in preparation for labor and delivery. Flexibility is particularly important in the hip and back joints, which tend to tighten up under the growing weight of the fetus and the shift in your center of gravity. As you learned in Chapter 3, the body's typical reaction to pain is to tighten up, which only makes the pain worse. If that happens during labor and delivery—if you tighten your pelvic floor muscles as a reaction to the pain—the baby is going to have a more difficult time passing through the vaginal canal, you'll have more pain, and you'll also face a greater risk of injuring the pelvic floor muscles, tissues, and nerves. So it's terribly important as a preparation for delivery to do the Letting Go program you learned back in Chapter 3—the exercises of Part 1 of the End-the-Pain routine—from deep breathing and the pelvic drop through all the stretches *except* the abdominals stretch.

The reason we exclude the abdominals stretch? Your abdomen is stretching all on its own, as the muscles make room for the growing fetus. Asking those muscles to stretch even more through exercise is not necessary.

Instead of the 11 exercises of Letting Go, therefore, do only 10. And if you find that it is just too tough, as your stomach expands, to do the butt stretch, do only nine of the exercises, excluding the butt stretch as well as the abdominals stretch.

It is never too late or too early to start practicing these tension-easing exercises. Whether you are in your first trimester or your last, a half hour of Letting Go stretching will stand you in good stead when those contractions start and you find yourself on the delivery table with your obstetrician or midwife telling you to "push" the baby out. These exercises will also help you feel more flexible—and therefore more comfortable—during the months of your pregnancy.

EASE YOUR DELIVERY: THE PREVENTIVE MASSAGE

Massaging the perineal body is an excellent way to prepare the vagina for delivery; it may make your time easier and less painful, and it can help prevent difficulties, complications, and injuries.

(Refer to Figure 1.3.) Start massaging the area at any time, but by all means begin a regular program of massage at least six weeks prior to delivery. At that time, you or your partner should start gently stretching the tissues at the vaginal opening as well. That means doing the internal pelvic massage you learned back in Chapter 5, only in this case, you're not probing for sore points, you're actually stretching the sides of the vagina outward and downward.

Lie on your back with a pillow or two behind your head and another under your upper back. Remember to visualize your pelvis as a clock on which your pubic bone is at the 12 o'clock position and the anus is at 6 o'clock. Insert the index fingers of both hands about an inch into the vagina at the 3 o'clock and 9 o'clock positions respectively. Gently stretch the sides of the vagina out and down. Hold the stretch for 20 seconds, then relax for 20 seconds. Do this three times, once a day, right up until delivery. It is excellent preparation for delivery, and it can help you avoid an episiotomy and prevent vaginal tears.

GAIN STRENGTH: THE KEGEL QUESTION

Just as important as relaxing the tension in your pelvic floor muscles and readying the tissue for delivery is strengthening the muscles. As discussed in Chapter 4, the key to strengthening the muscles of the pelvic floor is the Kegel, and many women wonder whether Kegels are appropriate during pregnancy. The answer is yes, with some qualifications.

It is true that the growth of the fetus puts extra pressure on the bladder, and this causes some increase in frequency of urination; it's a cliché that pregnant women are constantly in need of a bathroom. But this should not be seen as an invitation to just keep on doing Kegels. Moderation is needed. Here's the rule of thumb:

If you are *not leaking*, do 20 Kegels once or twice a week: 10 for two seconds, relaxing for two, 10 for 10 seconds, relaxing for 10 seconds. This will maintain your pelvic floor muscle strength without overworking the muscles.

If you *are leaking*, even just a little, do the 20 Kegel reps a few times a day—no more than three times—depending on the severity of the leaking. Again, hold the position for two seconds, relax for two, hold for 10 seconds, and relax for 10.

GAIN STRENGTH: MORE EXERCISES

Strengthening is essential to keep you fit during pregnancy, to smooth your delivery, and to make your return to normalcy fast and easy. These exercises keep your legs, upper back, and abdominals strong—and you'll be grateful for the results. (Once your baby is born and starts growing—fast—you'll be particularly grateful for that upper body strength.)

If you've been doing these exercises all along, start with 20 reps of each—30 if you can! If you're new to them, start off with 10 repetitions of each and work your way up. Remember to breathe and to rest between reps.

Pelvic Tilt

On your back, knees bent, feet flat and hip-width apart, tighten your abdominal muscles by sinking your belly button toward your spine—as if you were zipping up a tight pair of jeans—and tilt your pelvis upward toward the ceiling. Hold for 10 seconds, then relax for 10 seconds for one repetition. (Refer to p. 80 in Ch. 4; do with or without Kegels.) If you find it difficult to do the pelvic tilt during the last stages of pregnancy—if, like many women, lying on your back is uncomfortable or makes you short of breath—do the quadruped baby lift later in this section instead.

Squats

Stand with feet hip-width apart, feet forward of the line of your shoulders and slightly turned out. Tighten your abs. Slowly, on a count of three seconds, bend your knees as you lower your buttocks to a maximum of a 45-degree angle—or as close as possible. Lean forward slightly as you do this but keep your back straight—as if you were about to sit down on a chair. Make sure your knees don't go forward of the line of your toes. Rise back up to a standing position, also on a three-second count. Relax for five seconds. (Refer to p. 60 in Ch. 3.)

Bridge

Do this *only in the first four months of pregnancy.* After that, the fetus will be too big, and the exercise can decrease your blood flow as you lift.

Lie on your back with knees bent, feet flat and hip-width apart, arms at your sides. Tighten your abs. Slowly raise your pelvis. When you reach the top of the bridge, hold the position, then slowly lower the pelvis. Relax. (Refer to p. 57 in Ch. 3.)

Quadruped Baby Lift

Get down on all fours on your hands and knees. Hold your head in a straight line with your spine, with your chin tucked in. Keeping your back and neck straight, tighten your navel up to your spine, contracting your abs to "lift the baby." Hold for five seconds, relax for five seconds.

Quadruped Opposite Arm and Leg Raise

Still on all fours and holding the abdominal muscle tight, lift your left leg and right arm simultaneously while keeping your pelvis square to the floor. Hold for three seconds, then lower both arm and leg. Relax. Tighten the ab muscles again, and now raise your right leg and left arm. Hold for three seconds, lower, relax. (Refer to p. 59 in Ch. 3.)

Hip Adduction

On your back with your knees bent and feet hip-width apart, tighten your abs and squeeze a pillow or ball between your knees and hold the position for 10 seconds. Relax for 10 seconds. At the five-month marker, switch to doing this seated. (Refer to p. 79 in Ch. 4; do with or without Kegels.)

Hip External Rotation

On your back with your knees bent and feet together, tighten your abs and slowly separate your knees—feet still together—until the knees are about 24 inches apart. Add resistance by pressing your hands against the separating knees. (You may also use a resistance band.) Hold the position for three seconds and then slowly return your knees together in the center. Relax for five seconds. (Refer to p. 78 in Ch. 4; do with or without Kegels.) You can also perform this exercise in a seated position once you have reached five months.

HELPFUL HINTS

There's so much to think about during pregnancy that it's easy to forget some of the basics. While it's important to do the relaxation techniques and exercises in this chapter, it's also essential to keep up your cardiovascular routine as best you can—but be sure to monitor your comfort level and your breathing. If you find that your breathing is labored, slow down; if you feel discomfort or pain, cut back.

Posture is particularly important during pregnancy. Your bodily changes affect your stance and posture, and holding yourself upright of course gets more and more difficult as the fetus grows. Go back to Chapter 7 and practice the standing and seated posture exercises as often as you can. The better aligned you are, the less chance of injuring yourself, and the more strength you'll have for carrying your newborn.

Watch your body mechanics too. It's particularly important during pregnancy—mostly because of the shift in weight—to take care that you use your legs when you bend down to pick something up, not your back. Refer back to the photos on page 124 in Chapter 7, which demonstrate poor lifting and proper lifting. Be careful lowering yourself into a chair; hold on as you get seated. Slouching can be hard on the body, so stash a cushion behind your back when you're sitting down; it will support your posture.

If you have severe discomfort in your butt or low back region, give yourself the sore points massage you learned in Chapter 5. If that doesn't help, ask your health-care provider or physical therapist about using a sacroiliac support belt; these can be obtained from medical supply houses and are easily found via Internet search. This is a kind of splint that helps stabilize the pelvis and the sacroiliac joint, the joint below the spine that expands during pregnancy in order to accommodate a growing fetus. The belt effectively relieves pressure on the lower back and sacroiliac joint. However, it is essential to get a correct diagnosis from someone who specializes in pregnancy-related back pain.

Cushions can also help, both in easing the discomfort of lying down and in supporting your posture. As mentioned, you can use cushions to support your back, and try a cushion under the butt—to take away tailbone, pelvic, or sit bone pain.

Where nutrition is concerned, your doctor has certainly advised you about the best diet. But it's very important to avoid constipation, so keep away from the simple carbohydrates and from fried and high-fat foods, remember to eat fiber regularly, and refer back to Chapter 6 for a brush-up on ways to stay regular.

ONCE YOUR BABY IS BORN

Certainly you're eager to get back to your prepregnancy fitness level. The best way to do that is to keep up with the exercises and relaxation techniques described in this chapter—only more so: more reps, more resistance, more exercises. Obviously, don't start any exercise program until you have recouped fully from childbirth and have received approval from your doctor.

If you had a healthy vaginal delivery, your vaginal muscles and tissues have temporarily stretched, and Kegels are the best way to bring the muscles and tissue back to top form. But the rule of thumb is still operative: If you're leaking, do Kegels up to three times a day; if not, do them once or twice a week.

As to other exercise and certainly as regards your return to a cardiovascular routine, challenge yourself.

Some Precautions

There are exceptions, of course. The stretching of the abdominal muscles that occurred during pregnancy sometimes results in what's called a diastasis recti—an actual separation of the abdominal muscles. In due course, the separation is bridged naturally, and most of the time, the muscles will return to their prepregnancy closeness—but not always. So you can speed the process—or make it happen—by hugging your tummy as you do your pelvic tilts. Literally give yourself a hug—right below your ribs and above the pelvic bones, thus scrunching the muscles into a state approximating their normal, prepregnancy closeness. Hold the hug for 10 seconds, and do 10 reps twice a day.

After a couple weeks, add the more challenging abdominal exercises with the tummy hug, shown in Chapter 3, on pages 54–56. Also, abdominal binders specifically to help with this condition are available via the Internet.

If you suffered a vaginal tear, had an episiotomy, or delivered your baby via C-section, you will want to talk to your doctor about scar tissue mobilization—that is, a way of massaging either an internal or external scar, whichever your condition left you with, so that you don't get permanent adhesions that could produce pelvic floor dysfunction or lower abdominal pain. Ice can ease the discomfort in the initial stages. Ice the area for up to 15 minutes as many as five times a day to calm the painful nerve endings and any inflammation. Alternatively, you might want to do the contrast bath described in Chapter 7. Then ask your health-care provider how to do the scar tissue massage to prevent pelvic floor and abdominal muscle disorders.

CHAPTER 10

PELVIC FLOOR DISORDER IN CHILDREN

The first thing you should know about pelvic floor disorders in children is that they are not unusual.

If your child experiences urinary or fecal incontinence, urgency, frequency, and/or retention—that is, doesn't fully empty the bladder or bowels, or has trouble doing so—then he or she is not alone. Twenty percent of pediatrician visits are for incontinence. Some five million children complain of bed-wetting. Fifteen percent of pediatric appointments with gastrointestinal specialists are for lower bowel dysfunction. Clearly, pelvic floor disorders in children are not uncommon.

For the most part, younger children—those under the age of 10—will infrequently suffer pelvic pain, although some might feel the abdominal or rectal pain associated with constipation or lower abdominal pain due to urinary retention. Older children and teenagers, however, may experience the pain of tightened muscles or pelvic weakness, signals of the same disorders adults experience. This is not surprising, for indeed, the maturing muscles and tissue and bones of these older kids are subject to the same musculoskeletal issues as can affect grown-ups. After all, children have the same pelvic floor muscles we have; the muscles may simply be underdeveloped, or the child may be using the muscles incorrectly.

But although millions of kids suffer from these problems, often with consequences for the whole family's quality of life, few kids get the help they need—help that addresses the real underlying problem. Without such help, the psychological impact on the child can be substantial and very painful, with long-lasting influence. This chapter is about making sure that doesn't happen to your children—or to any children you know and care about.

THE CONDITIONS CHILDREN CAN SUFFER

Children today are typically fully toilet trained by the age of four. Most of the problems that occur between the ages of 4 and 10 therefore tend to be problems of incoordination—that is, instead of relaxing the pelvic floor muscles in order to void, the kid tightens up and "holds it in." Frequently, it's because something exciting is going on that the child doesn't want to miss. Heading for the nearest bathroom seems like a waste of time and a distraction—a chore of secondary importance. In due course, the inevitable happens: the child leaks stool or wets himself; there is involuntary excretion.

Sometimes, the cause is deeper. If toilet training was undertaken when the child was not ready for it, it can sometimes turn into a power struggle. If the power struggle persists, the child will continue to use the refusal to go to the bathroom as a weapon in the struggle.

Young children may also have issues that focus on the toilet itself: they might not feel comfortable in a strange toilet, or in one that looks unclean to them. I've known kids to express fear about the toilet itself, particularly the "scary" flushing that seems both loud and mysterious.

Sometimes, emotional distress from other causes gets expressed as a struggle over use of the toilet, and the child "holds it in" as a way of dealing with the distress. Discord between parents, illness or loss of a family member, even the worries over money or job security or world events that parents unwittingly transfer to their kids can all find their way to the bathroom, with incontinence or urgency, frequency or retention as the result.

As with adults, injury may also have an impact. A small tumble can be a big problem for a small child—especially if it injures the back, sacroiliac joint, or tailbone, and it can cause a pelvic floor disorder that will precipitate the symptoms kids find so embarrassing. By the same token, these symptoms may signal physical, sexual, or psychological abuse.

A fairly common condition in young kids is vesicoureteral reflux, in which the urine flows backwards from the bladder to the kidneys; the normal path is from the kidneys to the bladder to the urethra, from which it is excreted into the toilet. The condition can either be caused by or lead to chronic urinary tract infections, and it can result in scarring of and possible permanent damage to the kidneys. In this case, exercises like those in Chapter 3 that teach the child how to let go and how to stretch as well as the advice in the "Tips for the Toilet" section in Chapter 7 can help avoid urinary tract infections and other complications.

Whatever the particular condition the child experiences, and whatever the cause, any instance of pelvic floor disorder in children can qualify as a major medical problem, one that may affect the child's behavior and emotional health as well as family life as a whole—even eventually lead to severe psychosocial issues. As with grown-ups, children may feel the symptoms as life-limiting. They become embarrassed, ashamed, and anxious, may lose self-esteem, and typically shy away from such normal childhood activities as sports, playing with friends, and after-school activities.

But unlike adults, even teenagers, not to mention young children, find it difficult to understand what is happening to them physically and how their physical condition connects to their unhappiness. They can't understand why they are different from their friends. It's tough on the kids, and it's tough on the parents as well.

A CORRECT DIAGNOSIS IS KEY

How then should parents treat such disorders? The most important first step is to get a clear diagnosis of both the condition and, to the extent possible, the cause. For that, you will need to see a health-care professional—specifically, your child's pediatrician or a physical therapist trained in pediatric pelvic floor dysfunction.

But as with adults, as you read in the foreword to this book by Dr. Andrew Goldstein, it continues to be rare to find physicians who will consider musculoskeletal issues when they examine a patient—rarer still for physicians to prescribe the kind of natural healing advanced in this book. Unfortunately, giving a kid a pill may not be the answer for treating a problem of incontinence or retention; it doesn't always get to the root cause or address the source of the problem, and it can cause side effects and complications that can be further injurious to your child's health.

The solution to this dilemma? Make an appointment for your child with the pediatrician—and take this book with you. As a consumer of health-care services, you have the right to ask that musculoskeletal issues be addressed and that nonpharmaceutical therapies be considered. Your doctor may thank you in the end.

Of course there certainly *are* health-care providers—physicians, nurse practitioners, and physical therapists—who specialize in bladder and bowel disorders and/or who routinely address musculoskeletal disorders of the pelvic floor in children as well as in adults. Such professionals may apply a variety of techniques and therapies to treat the child.

Among these is therapeutic massage to be applied by trained professionals only, who will also likely prescribe home exercises like the ones in this book. Biofeedback has also proven to be particularly effective with children, who tend to respond well to this form of therapy. It is simply a noninvasive tool for showing children how to use their pelvic floor and abdominal muscles correctly to help with proper elimination. The kids literally reeducate the muscles, reteaching them to be coordinated. It's a very effective therapy for pelvic floor dysfunction in children, but again, it requires health-care providers fully trained in the technique.

WHAT YOU CAN DO AT HOME

Yes, there are things you can do at home to deal with your child's symptoms, mitigate his or her anxiety and embarrassment, and bolster his or her confidence.

Exercise and Massage

First of all, as with adults, if the problem is tightness or muscle incoordination, as evidenced in bladder or bowel retention or constipation, children can benefit from the relaxation exercises of the End-the-Pain routine in Chapter 3.

The abdominal massage and the lower extremity massage described in Chapter 5 can also help with issues of constipation and bladder or bowel retention. (Note: the internal massage in that chapter is absolutely off-limits for children; it is for sexually experienced and mature adults only.) For the abdominal massage in the case of constipation, ask the child to demonstrate how he or she can draw the letters ILU on his or her belly. Guide the demonstration, making sure the child is not going too fast and is applying sufficient pressure. Many kids enjoy having their parent do the massage for them; it's relaxing.

If the problem is muscle weakness leading to urinary or fecal incontinence—that is, if the child leaks—try the strengthening exercises of Chapter 4. To be sure, Kegels can be difficult to explain to a young child; this is one area, in fact, where biofeedback can be particularly useful.

Whether the issue is tightened muscles or weak muscles, if you're starting a routine of exercises and massage from Chapters 3, 4, and 5, be sure first to check your child's symptoms against the lists at the beginning of each chapter to make certain you're following the appropriate routine. Also, be sure that the child does no more than the number of repetitions called for.

The problem with kids and exercise is getting them to do it—consistently. That is really a parenting issue rather than a health issue, and how you deal with it will depend on your own style and your approach to discipline as well as on the child's age and temperament. In some cases, you'll need to adapt the exercises. For example, you might use a bubble-blower or a toy whistle to assist with the deep-breathing exercise. To use the toy whistle, ask the child to take a deep breath, and as he or she exhales, slowly count with the child to see how long he or she can keep the sound going. It's helpful also to have the child practice this while on the toilet.

It's great for kids to take control of their own problems, but incentives—like verbal encouragement and praise or even a system of material rewards—may be needed to get them going and to help them stick with it. One form of encouragement is to make a game of the exercises. For example, keep a record of how many repetitions the child does, then suggest that he or she try to beat the number the next day. Offering a reward for doing so provides further encouragement.

Another good idea is to do the exercises with your child; this shows support and can be a bonding experience. Try filling out the Symptoms Monitor in Chapter 2 with the child so that you can both keep track of progress.

Sometimes, however, kids may respond more readily to a professional than to a parent, especially if a power struggle is part of the problem. In such cases, it's advisable that an objective health-care provider monitor the child's exercise program.

Behavior and Lifestyle

In addition to the physical exercises, a program of behavior modification may be warranted—especially if the child is having emotional problems, isn't sleeping well, is acting out with eating issues, and the like. For that, it makes sense to consult a child psychologist or other mental health professional.

Many parents find it helpful to set a voiding schedule—for example requiring the child to go to the bathroom every two to three hours, depending on the amount the child drinks, as a way of regularizing excretion patterns and getting the child used to heading for the toilet routinely. Make sure the child is comfortable on the toilet seat—at least the one at home. Child-sized toilet seats work well; kids don't feel they are falling in. Put a stool under the child's feet to raise the knees above the hips; this relaxes the pelvic floor, facilitates bowel movement, and can make the child feel safer and more secure. Make sure the child doesn't run off the toilet to get back to play; this may result in incomplete emptying.

Nutrition

Nutrition can also be a useful tool in dealing with kids' pelvic floor disorders. If the child suffers from constipation, it's important to make sure he or she drinks plenty of water and eats plenty of fiber-rich foods. You may have to be creative with the fiber-rich foods, experimenting till you find those your child likes—certain high-fiber cereals, for example.

If frequency or leaking is the problem, make sure the child's diet is free of bladder irritants like soda, chocolate, or acidic or spicy foods. If the issue is abdominal bloating or pain, try eliminating dairy products for two weeks and see if the symptoms improve; if so, it may be an indication of lactose intolerance. During this dairyless time, you'll need to find other, nondairy foods that supply calcium to the child's diet. Again, consult Chapter 6 for more details on what your child should and should not eat to help with his or her problem.

In addition, be sure the child engages regularly in physical activity—sports, physical games, and the kind of kinetic play that comes so naturally to children. It's a great way to increase cardiovascular fitness, control weight, and strengthen the core, and of course, it's good for every child's overall health and sense of well-being.

CHAPTER 11

FOR MEN ONLY

Pelvic floor disorders aren't just a women's problem.

Although women do suffer disproportionately from pelvic floor disorders, dysfunction in this area of the body is by no means a "female issue." The pelvic floor is the pelvic floor, in men as in women. And while the genital anatomy and organs obviously differ between the two sexes, the pelvic floor muscles are the same, have the same purpose, function in almost the same exact way, and can malfunction with the same unhappy results. Moreover, the nerve pathways are the same in both sexes, although the names are slightly different, so nerve-related pain will radiate with the same cascading impact in men as in women.

There is, however, a strictly male-oriented component of pelvic floor disorder, and it is, unhappily, a not uncommon occurrence. That is, studies show that 95 percent of chronic prostatitis, pain in and around the prostate, is nonbacterial and very likely a result of pelvic floor dysfunction. "Nonbacterial" means that the pain is not a result of an infection or disease—and is therefore not treatable by antibiotics. Rather, such chronic nonbacterial prostatitis is a disorder of the muscles, nerves, or tissue; in other words, it is musculoskeletal in origin. It means that the urinary frequency, urgency, retention, and pain that men may feel in the urethra, bladder, abdomen, rectum, thigh, back, or genital region—pain that may afflict them when they walk, climb stairs, sit, lie down, void, or engage in sexual activity—may well be signs of this nonbacterial prostatitis. If that's the case, both the pain and its underlying cause are best addressed the natural way, with the exercises and other therapies detailed in this book—rather than with surgery or antibiotics.

I have treated a number of patients who were diagnosed with prostatitis and were prescribed antibiotics. After months of this pharmaceutical regimen—and no relief—they were finally referred for physical therapy and found both an end to their pain and a cure. Given what we keep learning about diseases that are resistant to antibiotics due to their overprescription and overuse, such experiences underlie the important object lesson of this book: make sure to ask your doctor if there isn't a noninvasive therapy for your pain or discomfort before you accept a recommendation of drugs or surgery. That is certainly the case when nonbacterial prostatitis is the diagnosis; it may well be cured with the exercises and therapies in this book without requiring drugs or the extreme measure of surgery.

WHAT CAUSES PELVIC FLOOR DISORDERS IN MEN?

Men typically suffer the same two basic categories of disorder that women suffer—namely, those that result from muscles and tissues that are too tight and/or from nerves that are irritated, and those that result from muscles that are too weak. Not surprisingly, the disorders derive from the same basic causes as well.

Maybe it was too many long, fast bike rides on that narrow, high-tech, Italian bicycle saddle. Maybe it was the heavy lifting you did when you helped out on your neighbor's house renovation, or decided you'd like to split the firewood logs yourself, or hauled the summer deck furniture back into the garage in the autumn, or took up weight training at the gym and did it to excess. A simple fall, especially if you landed on the tailbone, or that old sports injury from when you slid into third base last summer and hammered your sacroiliac joint: any and all of these can result, sooner or later, in a pelvic floor disorder.

Of course, acute prostatitis is another cause of pelvic floor disorder in men. A diagnosis of chronic nonbacterial prostatitis is typically the spasming, tightening, and shortening of the pelvic floor muscle. In the case of acute prostatitis when antibiotics are necessary, the irritation and discomfort that it produces can lead to a habitual holding and tightening of the pelvic floor muscles. Result? Pelvic floor dysfunction and its accompanying pain.

One other cause that happens to men only is a prostatectomy—that is, the removal of the prostate—or radiation treatment for prostate cancer or such other reproductive cancers as testicular cancer. As any prostate cancer patient knows, these therapies for the disease can result in problems of incontinence and erectile dysfunction. In such cases, your oncologist may only be able to promise you that function will come back "within a year or so," not a terribly cheerful prognosis. What your doctor may not tell you is that a specialist in pelvic floor dysfunction may be able to help. So will the exercises and other therapies in this book. Follow them, and you may well speed your recovery and avoid problems in the future.

GENTLEMEN, HERE'S HOW TO HEAL YOUR PELVIC FLOOR DISORDER

Typically, the disorders deriving from tight, spasmed muscles can cause urinary and bowel urgency, frequency, and retention; tension and pain throughout the pelvic, abdominal, genital, back, and hip regions; and pain and dysfunction associated with urination, defecation, or sexual activity. These disorders can be addressed with the End-the-Pain exercise routine in Chapter 3 along with the massage therapies in Chapter 5.

Men also suffer from pelvic floor weakness and may experience the incontinence, decreased libido, and erectile dysfunction that may be the result from such weakness. And while we tend not to think of men doing Kegels, they can and do—the same way that women do them with outcomes as beneficial as those women experience. After all, men certainly have sexual muscles—specifically, the PC muscle—and strengthening it through Kegels and other exercises can greatly enhance sexual activity, pleasure, and longevity in men as in women. Refer to Chapter 4 for those exercises.

In addition to the exercises, men will also benefit from following the recommendations in these pages for self-care, nutrition, and other natural healing therapies.

CHAPTER 12

THE NATURAL WAY TO HEAL PELVIC PAIN

Everyone knows what to do if they sprain an ankle. It's almost automatic. Stop moving, put your foot up, ice it if you can, and take an ibuprofen. If, after a couple of days, all that doesn't reduce the swelling, lessen the pain, and make it possible for you to stand and walk, that's when you go see your orthopedist or physical therapist.

Or suppose you lean over to lift a heavy box from the floor, or to move the armchair, or to pick up your baby from the crib, and—ouch!—your back goes out. Again, you know what to do: bend your knees and straighten up slowly, apply ice, rest as best you can, and pop an over-the-counter pill. Again, in most cases, that will do it, but if not, you know to go to an orthopedist or physical therapist for relief.

But when you suddenly feel that you will not make it to a bathroom in time, so severe is your urinary urgency, or when you feel a pain in your pelvic area but can't quite pinpoint where, or when you feel bloated and uncomfortable and as if you are straining to move your bowels, you're not sure what to do to find relief. Your first thought is probably that you have a bacterial infection in some internal organ. Or you might rush to the Internet to check out your symptoms and look for a diagnosis. A disorder in your pelvic floor muscles is probably the last thing most people think of.

Yet a musculoskeletal disorder—that is, a problem in the muscles, connective tissue, nerves, or in your body's alignment—is a likely cause of your pain, as you have now learned. You also now know that your pain can be relieved and your condition healed through the natural healing of this book—the exercises, massage, nutrition, self-care, and relaxation techniques you've been learning and practicing.

Does this mean that traditional medicine has no role in your recovery? On the contrary. For one thing, it is vitally important that you work with a health-care provider who can ensure the diagnosis, track your symptoms, and monitor your recovery—so long as you find the *right* health-care provider. That means a doctor, physical therapist, nurse, or other professional who specializes in pelvic floor dysfunction and pelvic pain.

Under no circumstances does it mean, however, that you should turn to the Internet. Like most health-care professionals, I despair at what patients do to themselves when they self-diagnose and self-medicate as a result of Internet searches. Five patients with the same disorder will come up with five different Internet diagnoses and courses of treatment; all will probably do themselves more harm than good.

Use the Internet—and specifically, the Websites listed in Appendix B of this book—to find a health-care professional who specializes in pelvic pain, but please do not use it to treat your condition. You may cause yourself real injury—physically and/or emotionally—if you do so.

WHAT CAN TRADITIONAL MEDICINE DO?

Certainly, medical interventions can be helpful for certain disorders in certain patients. It must be understood, however, that medication *alone* cannot provide a cure for musculoskeletal disorders. Moreover, medication can produce side effects, and you and your health-care practitioner will want to weigh the impact of those side effects against the benefits.

This is why it is so important to find a health-care practitioner who is an expert in pelvic floor disorders. Only such expertise can be relied on if you are going to obtain an accurate and precise diagnosis of your disorder.

In addition, you should never be afraid to ask for a second opinion. If you feel that a course of treatment "sounds wrong," or if a prescription or recommendation doesn't seem to be working, by all means go to another practitioner and get another examination. This is especially true if surgery is recommended; a second or even a third opinion is really essential.

Once you have a diagnosis, there are any number of medical interventions possible. Here are just a few of them:

- Muscle relaxants to help relax the pelvic floor and surrounding muscles
- Anti-inflammatories to help rid the body of inflammation
- Antidepressants or antiseizure medications to calm both peripheral and centralized nerve pain
- Medications for organ pain—for example, bladder pain
- Medications to normalize bladder and/or bowel function
- Topical creams to relieve vaginal or rectal skin irritations or disorders
- Hormone therapy if a hormone imbalance is diagnosed.

In many cases, you'll need to give the medication a couple of months to work. If you're considering stopping a course of medication, don't do it "cold turkey"; wean yourself from the medication under the guidance of your health-care practitioner. Keep in mind also that it is possible for the body to become accustomed to a medication, in which case it may lose its efficacy; you may then need to increase the dose or switch to another medication.

In addition to these medications, your referring health-care provider may suggest nerve blocks to calm nerve pain, trigger point injections to relieve muscular spasms, or Botox to help relax the pelvic floor muscles so that you can lengthen them through the massage techniques of Chapter 5.

In the event that your doctor or other practitioner refers you for psychological counseling, cognitive behavioral therapy has proven to be particularly effective in helping patients deal with the pain and stress of pelvic floor disorders. If acupuncture is prescribed, dry needling into the trigger points has been demonstrated to be most beneficial. Hypnosis may also help assuage pain by helping change the way the brain processes pain signals. Yoga, specifically the gentler forms of practice, has been shown to be very helpful in calming the nervous system and diminishing the pain of pelvic floor disorder.

None of these interventions should be a substitute for the therapies in this book, but all may prove to be useful supplements or complements when recommended—I'll say it one more time—by a health-care professional experienced in treating pelvic floor disorders.

HELPING THE HEALING

In the decade in which I've been specializing in treating pelvic floor dysfunction, I have helped literally thousands of patients. That is a lot of people, and I have seen a lot of pain and suffering.

I have also seen thousands of patients recover from pelvic floor dysfunction. I have watched as their pain diminished and disappeared, and as they once again resumed full, normal functioning—often, better than before.

But it takes time. Improvement may come slowly and in small increments. If you undertake the healing therapies in this book and find that your disorder is diminishing and your pain is subsiding, it means you are on the right track. Keep going.

If you find you are impatient over the pace of your progress—for example, if you've been at it for months with little improvement—consult with your health-care practitioner. You may need something else to get you to where you want to be.

Stress reduction is an essential component of the healing process. Time and again, I have seen that if you have two patients with a similar diagnosis, the patient who works at reducing his or her stress will have a faster recovery and better result than the one who does not. This demonstrable reality is being increasingly confirmed by laboratory studies and statistical data across the medical profession; stress slows healing.

Another thing I've noticed that can really make a difference is a positive attitude. That's tough to have when you're in agony, and I know that the pain of pelvic floor disorder can often be real agony. But if you can see the light at the end of the tunnel, if you know that what you are doing really will bring about change, attitude can go a long way toward helping you heal.

I've noticed also that patients who do the whole program—all the therapies of this book—heal most effectively. Their recoveries are faster and more complete than for those patients who do only the exercises, for example, or pay attention only to the self-massage techniques. Doing it all is best, and daunting as the prospect may seem, an inclusive regimen soon becomes habit—something you do automatically, without thinking about it.

Many patients, in fact, have used the therapies in this book as a mere starting-point for creating life routines that combine exercise, relaxation, and healthy eating in creative ways. So don't feel restricted by my recommendations. If you find that yoga helps your symptoms, that watching a movie relaxes your mind and body, that meditation equates to emotional support, or that you need to take a "mental health" break every other hour, do it. Whatever works for you is worth integrating into your life for a lifetime.

After all, the key is not just to end the pain and heal the disorder. The aim is to be healthy at the core for life. I hope you'll agree that such a goal is worth the effort of these techniques and therapies for natural healing.

DISORDERS OF THE PELVIC FLOOR: SIGNS AND SYMPTOMS, CONSEQUENCES, AND CAUSES

SIGNS AND SYMPTOMS

Musculoskeletal Dysfunction Resulting in or from Pelvic Floor Disorders

Pelvic floor disorders commonly result in a referral pain pattern—that is, the pain radiates into the low back, thighs, and into the suprapubic, abdominal, and pelvic region. The pain may start in one small area, but because the pain persists (and usually for a prolonged period of time), it may cause hypersensitivity and can spread to any or all of the above-mentioned referral areas. Persistent pain may cause increased sensitivity in the local nerves and could potentially spread to the central nervous system (called central sensitization). Here are some of the common musculoskeletal dysfunctions that result in or from pelvic disorders:

Low Back/Sacroiliac Dysfunction. General low back pain can be caused by trunk stabilizer weakness, by possible malalignments of the lumbar spine, pelvis, and sacrum, or by various dysfunctions in the vertebrae and discs. Poor body mechanics and prolonged sitting may aggravate the condition.

Sacral Pain. Ligamentous laxity (ligaments that are lax or overstretched from malalignment of the sacroiliac joint), muscle imbalance, and postural strains can cause sacral pain. Abnormal sacral function usually presents as pain on one side more than the other.

Groin or Pubic Pain. Adductor muscle strains, pelvic floor referred pain, or ligamentous laxity of the pubic symphysis (which is where the pubic bones of the pelvis join below the abdominal muscles) can lead to groin or pubic pain. Pain may increase with walking and transitional movements.

Piriformis Syndrome. Persistent, severe radiating pain extending from the sacrum to the hip, gluteal region, and posterior upper leg may be due to piriformis shortening and spasming. The piriformis muscle connects the sacrum to the hip joint and is a hip external rotator.

Iliopsoas Syndrome. Spasm of the iliopsoas muscle may produce pain in the lower abdomen, low back, or pelvic floor. The pain pattern can be similar to that of appendicitis, ovarian problems, or bowel disorders. The iliopsoas muscle connects the low back and pelvic bone to the thighbone.

Any of the above-mentioned dysfunctions can result in, or contribute to, pelvic floor dysfunction. If the dysfunction results in one side tightening or spasming, it can result in a dysfunction in the lumbopelvic region. For example, one side of the pelvic bone could rotate, resulting in abnormal tension in some of the pelvic floor muscles and nerves. The dysfunction could also result in tightening or spasming in certain muscles to compensate for the malalignment.

Pelvic Floor Pain, Tension, and Nerve Involvement in Both Men and Women

Pelvic Congestion. The pelvic veins are susceptible to chronic dilatation, which results in venostasis (the blood accumulates in the veins and doesn't flow), resulting in venous congestion of the pelvic veins. Signs and symptoms of pelvic congestion include chronic pelvic pain, dyspareunia, urinary frequency, urgency and/or retention, infertility, erectile dysfunction, and possible back and leg pain. Patients may complain of a dull ache that is aggravated by physical activity (especially with standing).

Pelvic congestion may require lymphedema therapy to improve circulation and the venostasis.

Pudendal Neuralgia. The pudendal nerve originates from the sacral plexus (S2–S4). It has both sensory and motor fibers. The sensory pudendal nerve branches into three smaller nerves: the inferior rectal nerve (which supplies part of the rectum and the surrounding skin), the perineal nerve (which supplies the perineum, vagina, male scrotum, labia, and urethra), and the dorsal nerve of the clitoris or penis. The motor branch of the nerve supplies the external anal sphincter, sphincter muscles of the bladder, and the muscles of the pelvic floor. Neuralgia—that is, irritation or pain— in the distribution of the pudendal nerve may result in sensory symptoms in any or all areas it supplies and may cause spasms in the muscles. A common site for pudendal nerve irritation may be at the Alcock's canal and/or at the obturator internus muscle. The sensory symptoms could manifest as itching, burning, tingling, cold sensations, and pain. The sensory symptoms may extend into the groin, abdomen, legs, and buttocks.

Signs and symptoms of pudendal neuralgia may include the following:

- Pelvic pain with sitting, but improvement with standing or sitting on a toilet seat
- Discomfort with tight clothing
- Bladder and/or bowel symptoms (hesitancy, frequency, retention, constipation, IBS-like symptoms)
- Dyspareunia and/or pain or spasm after orgasm
- Possible abnormal pudendal nerve motor latency test

Peripheral Nerve Pain Referrals. If any of the following nerves are irritated, the pain can be referred as follows:

- The genitofemoral nerve refers to upper part of the front of the thigh and slightly below the pubic bone.
- The ilioinguinal nerve refers to the inner thigh and the lateral part of the perineum.
- The iliohypogastric nerve refers to lower abdomen, groin, and lateral part of the perineum.
- The lateral femoral cutaneous nerve refers to the lateral and front of the thigh.
- The posterior femoral cutaneous nerve refers to the perineum, gluteal region, and the back of the thigh and leg.
- The obturator nerve refers from the groin area down the inner thigh area.
- The superior hypogastric and inferior hypogastric plexus and the ganglion impar are bundles of nerves, and they both are a part of the sympathetic nervous system. The sympathetic nervous system helps control stress, so if these bundles are affected, it can be difficult to control heart rate, and pain can be referred to the pelvic floor area.

Tension Myalgia of the Pelvic Floor. This term is used to consolidate various pelvic floor syndromes, including the following:

- **Pelvic pain.** Pain in the lower abdominal and pelvic region can be caused by changes in the muscles, nerves, or other tissues. Trigger points can be formed in and may refer to the pelvic floor, abdomen, back, hip, or leg region.
- **Coccydynia.** Pain in and around the region of the coccyx bone or tailbone is called coccydynia. It may involve the pelvic floor muscles, the coccygeus muscle, and/or the gluteus maximus muscle.
- **Levator ani syndrome.** This syndrome involves pain, pressure, or ache in the sacrum, coccyx, rectum, and pelvic diaphragm that may increase with intercourse, sitting, defecation, and constipation. Pain may refer to the thigh, coccyx/sacrum, or gluteal region. Severe, sharp burning or aching with urination may also occur, caused by unusual tension in the levator ani muscles.
- **Proctalgia fugax.** This is a spasm of the puborectalis muscle causing flatulence, difficult and painful defecation, and sharp, fleeting rectal pain lasting seconds to several hours.
- **Anismus.** This is an inability to penetrate the rectum due to spasmed muscles such as internal and external anal sphincters and the levator ani muscles. It causes increased difficulty when voiding and leads to constipation.
- **Hemorrhoids.** Pelvic floor muscle weakness, constipation, straining during bowel movements, and excessive straining during delivery can all result in hemorrhoids.

In Women Only

Pelvic Inflammatory Disease (PID). PID involves infection and inflammation in the pelvic cavity, particularly of the female reproductive organs. It can cause scarring around the fallopian tubes, which can lead to infertility, pelvic pain, and other problems. PID includes endometritis, salpingitis, peritonitis, and more.

Endometriosis. Endometriosis is a medical condition in which tissue similar to uterine tissue is found outside the uterus (often in the ovaries and/or fallopian tubes). The tissue can also be found in scars (from a C-section or laparoscopy, for example) and on the bladder, bowel, intestines, colon, appendix, and rectum. Rarely, it is found inside the vagina and bladder or on the skin. There is no known cause of endometriosis, but it is believed that estrogen exacerbates the condition, and regulation of estrogen production is the medical option for endometriosis treatment. The most common symptom of endometriosis is pelvic pain, which is often debilitating. Other symptoms include dyspareunia, fatigue, painful urination, painful bowel movements, and such other gastrointestinal problems as bloating and abdominal cramps. Diagnosis of endometriosis is through laparoscopy and biopsy of the abnormal tissue.

Vulvodynia (Vulvar Pain). Vulvodynia is the medical term for chronic vulvar discomfort. It is characterized by burning, irritation, rawness, dull or achy pain, and typically, inability to have vaginal penetration without pain.

Vaginismus. This is the medical term denoting inability to penetrate the introitus, or vaginal opening, due to muscle spasms of the superficial and/or deep pelvic floor muscles. Symptoms include dyspareunia and difficulty inserting a tampon or a speculum during a gynecological exam.

Vulvar Vestibulitis. Symptoms of vulvar vestibulitis include severe pain on vestibular touch or vaginal entry and erythema (redness) in the vestibule and Bartholin's gland openings.

Dyspareunia. This is the medical term for painful intercourse, which can be divided into pain upon initial vaginal penetration or with deep penetration. Trigger points and/or connective tissue restrictions within the superficial muscles and fascia of the perineum or scar tissue within the perineal body can cause initial penetration pain. Pain with deep penetration can be caused by spasms of the levator ani, obturator internus, coccygeus, and/or iliopsoas muscles.

Menstrual Pain and Disorders. Dysmenorrhea and endometriosis-related menstrual pain may be located in the pelvic region and lower abdominal area and result in significant tightness of the iliopsoas, lumbosacral, and pelvic floor muscles due to chronic pain holding patterns.

Herpetic Neuralgia. The HPV virus irritates the nerves and neural pathways, and as a result, the pelvic floor muscles can get irritated and tighten. Symptoms include tingling, twitching, burning, shooting pain, numbness, or aching pain.

Skin Conditions. There are several skin conditions that can cause pelvic pain:

- **Lichen planus.** Symptoms include inflammation and itching due to skin lesions; scarring and adhesions may lead to narrowing of the vagina.
- **Lichen sclerosus.** This is a chronic skin eruption diagnosed with biopsy; lesions are associated with itching and burning and painful intercourse.

In Men Only

Prostatitis. Prostatitis is any type of inflammation of the prostate gland. In 1999, the National Institutes of Health identified prostatitis in four different categories:

- **Acute bacterial prostatitis.** This involves an acute infection of the urinary tract. Symptoms include fever, chills, pain in the low back and genital area, body aches, urinary frequency, nocturia (nighttime frequency), painful urination (typically burning), and possible penile discharge. See your health-care provider immediately for antibiotic treatment if you suspect you have this condition.

- **Chronic bacterial prostatitis.** This is a recurrent infection of the prostate. It is rare, occurring in less than 5 percent of patients. The symptoms mimic intermittent acute bacterial prostatitis. The treatment is a prolonged course of antibiotics. Men with this condition may require physical therapy if antibiotics don't help. Recurrent infections may be caused by incomplete urinary evacuation (from a neurogenic bladder or from benign prostatic hypertrophy) or by prostatic stones.

- **Chronic nonbacterial prostatitis/chronic pelvic pain syndrome (CPPS)/pelvic myoneuropathy.** Men with these conditions may or may not have inflammation. Symptoms include discomfort or pain in the pelvic region (at least three months), which may radiate from the back to the rectum to the tip of the penis, with possible voiding and sexual symptoms. The person may have difficulty sitting due to the pain and discomfort. Antibiotics typically do not help with this diagnosis. These conditions may be a result of myofascial pain syndrome or neurogenic (nerve) inflammation. Treatment includes physical and behavioral therapy.

- **Asymptomatic inflammatory prostatitis.** Typically, a person with this condition has no genitourinary symptoms, but higher levels of white blood cells have been identified during evaluation. Prostate cancer needs to be ruled out through a PSA (prostate-specific antigen) test given by your urologist.

Prostatodynia or Chronic Pelvic Pain Syndrome (CPPS). These terms are used to designate unexplained complaints of chronic pelvic pain associated with either (1) nonspecific voiding symptoms and/or pain located in or around the groin, genitalia, or perineum, or (2) the absence of pus and bacteria in the urine, with or without excess white cells or bacteria, on results from tests of the prostate fluid in male patients.

Bladder Disorders in Both Men and Women

The common symptoms of bladder abnormality include urinary frequency (greater than one bathroom trip for every two awake hours); urgency, hesitancy and/or retention; nocturia (nighttime urinary frequency: more than one trip to the bathroom in the night); pain in the urethra, bladder, and/or pelvis; pressure, spasming, or difficulty with initiating urination; and/or a weak urine stream and/or a stream that stops and starts.

Interstitial Cystitis (IC). Also known as painful bladder syndrome (PBS), interstitial cystitis presents as recurring pain or discomfort in the bladder and the surrounding pelvic region. Signs and symptoms may include urinary urgency, frequency, or retention; dyspareunia; pain in the back, suprapubic area, and/or abdomen; nocturia (nighttime urinary frequency); and pain before, during, or after urination. It may also result in incontinence.

Urethral Syndrome. This involves urethral pain, burning, and sensitivity.

Urgency-Frequency Syndrome. This disorder causes urinary frequency, urgency, hesitancy, or retention with or without pain in the bladder, urethra, abdomen, or pelvis.

In the case of all of these bladder symptoms, irritation in the lining of the bladder or urethra can also irritate surrounding tissues, including skeletal muscle tissue. If this irritation persists and continues to irritate the surrounding muscles, trigger points can result. Trigger points result in increased tightening and shortening of the muscle, which can create more pain, irritation, and musculoskeletal imbalance.

Frequent trips to the bathroom when the bladder is not completely full can result in confusing or incorrect messages being sent to and from the brain and the bladder.

This may occur because the bladder feels irritated, and thus the person tries to get relief by going to the bathroom. Then the bladder develops a mind of its own, and it starts to give off false signals.

In response to these frequent trips to the bathroom, the person may try to "hold it in." This results in tightening of the pelvic floor muscles. Chronic or continuous tightening of any muscles will result in the muscles shortening; in so doing, the muscles tighten around the bladder, and this produces the feeling of having to urinate even when the bladder is not full. Thus the vicious circle continues. Bladder disorders as a result of musculoskeletal dysfunction can be helped through physical therapy.

Bowel Disorders in Both Men and Women

The common symptoms of bowel abnormality include bowel frequency, urgency, and/or retention; gas; diarrhea; constipation; bloating; rectal and/or abdominal pain, pressure, or spasm; difficulty with initiation; and/or incontinence.

Constipation. Defined as delayed or abnormal colonic transport, constipation may result from tight and/or weakened pelvic floor and abdominal musculature. Constipation as a result of muscle dysfunction can be managed conservatively with physical therapy. Treatment consists of bowel stimulation through abdominal massage and trigger point release.

The use of oral contraceptive pills at puberty affects colon motility adversely and may lead to problems with constipation.

Diarrhea. It is defined as the passage of an increased amount of feces. Chronic diarrhea (diarrhea that lasts more than three weeks) is a symptom of irritable bowel syndrome, Crohn's disease, and ulcerative colitis, and it can be caused by some medications.

Medications that cause diarrhea include digoxin, laxatives, antacids, certain antimicrobial agents, thiazide diuretics, and alcohol. Antidiarrheal drugs include Imodium and Lomotil.

Inflammatory Bowel Disease (IBD). This group includes Crohn's disease and ulcerative colitis. Crohn's disease is an inflammation of the digestive tract (anywhere from mouth to anus). It can affect all layers of the intestine and most commonly affects the small intestine (ileum). Ulcerative colitis is an inflammation of the top layer of the lining of the large intestine (colon and rectum). The inflammation can result in ulcers in the top layer. Signs and symptoms of both may include abdominal pain, diarrhea, rectal bleeding, weight loss, fever, arthritis, and skin problems.

Irritable Bowel Syndrome (IBS). IBS encompasses a group of symptoms that represent the most common disorder of the gastrointestinal system. Signs and symptoms of IBS may include abdominal pain or discomfort, bloating, gas, and such changes in bowel pattern as more frequent bowel movements, diarrhea, and/or constipation.

All of these disorders can result in increased toxins in the gut, which irritates surrounding tissues, including skeletal muscle tissue. If this irritation persists, trigger points can result. Trigger points lead to increased tightening and shortening of the muscle, which can create more pain and irritation. Also, the spasming of the intestinal smooth muscle (which can result from any bowel disorder) can also irritate the surrounding tissue and result in spasming of the skeletal muscle. Chronic straining can also result in overloading and strain of the skeletal muscle and surrounding tissues.

As with bladder dysfunction, any bowel disorder may result in abdominal and pelvic floor muscle and tissue tightening and trigger points as a response to the pain or discomfort, thereby worsening the pain or discomfort. Pain also may be felt in the lower back, leg, and buttocks area.

Musculoskeletal dysfunctions caused by IBS, constipation, and the other bowel disorders can be treated with physical therapy through abdominal, back, gluteal, and pelvic floor myofascial trigger point release.

CONSEQUENCES OF PELVIC FLOOR WEAKNESS

Pelvic Organ Prolapse

Weak pelvic floor musculature or chronic straining can produce a feeling of "falling out" or fullness. Both men and women may suffer a prolapse of the rectum into the posterior pelvic floor wall. In addition, women can suffer the following prolapses:

- **Cystocele.** Descent of the bladder downward and backward into the anterior vaginal wall.
- **Uterine prolapse.** Uterine cervix descent causing vaginal vault descent.
- **Urethrocele.** Descent of the urethra in the anterior vaginal wall.
- **Enterocele.** Displacement of the pouch of Douglas into the posterior vaginal wall.

Incontinence

Urinary stress incontinence is involuntary urine loss due to an increase in abdominal pressure, such as coughing, sneezing, lifting, or running. Urinary urge incontinence is involuntary urine loss due to a strong desire to urinate (urgency), with only a quick warning. With mixed incontinence, both urge and stress incontinence are combined.

In addition, pelvic floor disorder may lead to fecal incontinence, the involuntary loss of fecal matter or gas, and/or staining of underwear caused by either weak or hypertonic (tight) pelvic floor muscles or by poor toileting habits.

Sexual Dysfunction

In both men and women, pelvic floor disorders and the resulting weakness of the muscles can cause decreased libido or difficulty or inability to reach orgasm. Decreased libido can also be caused by hormonal imbalance, medications (for example, as a side effect of antidepressants), or decreased blood flow or congestion as from pelvic congestion.

In addition, both men and women can experience pain during or after sexual activity. Women may also complain of pain with the initial penetration, in deep penetration, with thrusting, and from lack of lubrication. Dyspareunia may be due to superficial scarring, adhesions, skin or nerve irritation, or muscle tenderness or tightness.

Men may suffer erectile dysfunction, the persistent failure to achieve and sustain erections of sufficient rigidity during sexual activity. This may be secondary to pelvic floor muscle tension, weakness, or pelvic congestion, or it could result from pain during or after intercourse.

CAUSES OF PELVIC FLOOR DISORDER

There are a variety of causes of pelvic floor disorders:

- Weakness in trunk and pelvic stabilizers, and possible malalignments of the lumbar spine, sacroiliac joint, and pelvis, resulting in muscle imbalance and possible muscle shortening
- Poor body mechanics or poor posture
- Chronic inflammatory conditions: prostatitis, cystitis, endometriosis, pelvic inflammatory disease (PID), colitis, inflammatory bowel disorder (IBD), and others
- Infections: urinary tract infection, yeast infection, bacterial infection

- Chronic holding patterns that develop because of ongoing stress, childhood or domestic abuse (physical, sexual, or verbal), premature or traumatic toileting, or abnormal bladder or bowel habits
- Trauma: a fall onto the tailbone or sacrum (lower back region), traumatic childbirth, abuse
- Repetitive motion or patterned habits causing strain on the pelvic floor muscles and possible microtrauma to the tissues (First causes might include repetitive heavy lifting, chronic straining of the bowels or bladder, and such physical activities as Pilates, ballet, swimming, and playing wind instruments.)
- Referred pain from other pain areas, such as visceral pain
- Muscle incoordination in the pelvis and possibly in the abdomen—for example, from contracting the pelvic floor muscles when trying to evacuate, instead of relaxing the muscles
- Sustained positions for prolonged periods of time
- Skin conditions: lichen sclerosus, lichen planus, and more
- Pelvic floor muscle weakness due to disuse, injury, or chronic straining

Postsurgical Conditions

In men, a prostatectomy and bladder replacement for postcancer treatment can aggravate pelvic floor disorder.

The following can both give rise to and aggravate pelvic floor disorder in women:

- **C-section.** May result in abdominal weakness, low back pain, scar adhesions, poor posture, and poor body mechanics as well as visceral dysfunction.
- **Hysterectomy.** A vaginal or abdominal procedure that may result in scar adhesions, and /or tension or weakness in the pelvic floor, abdomen, or hip flexor.

- **Episiotomy.** Vaginal tearing during childbirth leading to scar adhesions, pelvic floor muscle weakness, pain, and dyspareunia.
- **Laparoscopy.** Abdominal and visceral scar adhesions.

Any of these conditions may result in bladder, bowel, and/or sexual dysfunction with or without dysfunction of the pelvic floor muscles. Any incision into muscle results in weakness in the muscle and possibly in adjacent muscles.

FACTORS THAT MAY IMPEDE OR DELAY HEALING

Healing of pelvic floor disorder can be hindered by a number of factors:

- **Diet.** Certain foods and beverages can aggravate symptoms.
- **Constipation.** Puts extra pressure on pelvic floor, abdominal, and back muscles, while straining exacerbates the condition.
- **Any noxious stimuli.** Healing cannot proceed while irritation persists.
- **Muscular dysfunction.** Restrictions, tightness, or trigger points in the pelvic floor or surrounding muscles and connective tissue.
- **Skeletal malalignment.** Resulting in muscle imbalance or pinched nerve delays recovery.
- **Incoordination of the pelvic floor and abdominal muscles.** Inability to use pelvic floor and abdominal muscles correctly and efficiently.
- **Stress or such emotional/psychological disorders as depression, anxiety, bipolar disorder, etc.** Decreases body's immune system, can exacerbate pain and excite the nervous system.

- **Hormonal imbalances.** Among other impacts, may adversely affect tissue elasticity, making healing more difficult.
- **Coexisting illnesses.** Compromise the body's immune system, burdening the healing process.
- **Sleep disturbance.** The body uses sleep for tissue and organ recovery; sleep disturbance retards that process.
- **Participating in activities that tend to exacerbate the patient's symptoms.** For example, if sitting increases your pain, then you need to limit it until you are healed. Similarly, sexual activity may increase symptoms; therefore, you may need to limit sexual activity until you are healed.
- **Pain that fluctuates—for example, menstrual pain.** Results in a continued pain cycle that may discourage the patient.

The majority of the disorders presented in this appendix can be ameliorated or cured by following the appropriate program and guidelines in this book. See a health-care provider who specializes in pelvic floor dysfunction for a proper diagnosis. Refer to the resources in Appendix B to help you find a provider.

RESOURCES

WEBSITES

Most of the websites below can direct you to an appropriate health-care provider. Some of the sites do not provide street addresses, but there is typically an e-mail address where you can direct a question.

American Physical Therapy Association: www.apta.org (Click "Find a PT" and select "Women's Health" in the "Expertise" box.)
Biofeedback Certification Institute of America: www.bcia.org
Endometriosis Association: endometriosisassn.org
International Foundation for Functional Gastrointestinal Disorders: iffgd.org
International Pelvic Pain Society: pelvicpain.org
International Urogynecological Association: iuga.org
Interstitial Cystitis Association: ichelp.org
Interstitial Cystitis Network: ic-network.com
Irritable Bowel Association: ibsassociation.org
National Lymphedema Network: lymphnet.org
National Vulvodynia Association: nva.org
Prostatitis Association: prostatitis.org

Psychology Resource: psychology.com
Society for Pudendal Neuralgia: spuninfo.org
The Women's Sexual Health Foundation: twshf.org

The following websites can give you more information regarding pelvic floor dysfunction, pelvic pain, and chronic pain syndromes:

beyondbasicsphysicaltherapy.com
painchannel.com
hisandherhealth.com

Support groups exist for just about every pelvic floor diagnosis, so search on your particular symptoms to find the appropriate website; you're likely to find chat rooms and patient support groups.

BOOKS

Carter, Mark, and Lisa Carter. *Completely Overcome Vaginismus: The Practical Approach to Pain-Free Intercourse*. Vaginismus. com, 2002.

Daniluk, Judith C, and Sandra R. Leiblum. *Women's Sexuality Across the Life Span*. New York: Gilford Press, 1998.

Goldstein, Andrew, M.D., and Marianne Brandon, Ph.D. *Reclaiming Desire: 4 Keys to Finding Your Lost Libido*. Emmaus, Penn.: Rodale, 2004.

Howard, Fred M., M.D., Paul J. Perry, M.D., James Carter, M.D., and Ahmed M. El-Minawi, M.D. *Pelvic Pain: Diagnosis and Management*. Philadelphia: Lippincott Williams & Wilkins, 2000.

Hulme, Janet A. *Bladder and Bowel Issues for Kids*. Montana: Phoenix Publishing, 2003.

————. *Geriatric Incontinence: A Behavioral and Exercise Approach to Treatment.* Missoula, Mont.: Phoenix Publishing, 1999.

————. *Pelvic Pain & Low Back Pain: A Handbook for Self Care & Treatment.* Missoula, Mont.: Phoenix Publishing, 2002.

Hutcherson, Hilda, M.D. *Pleasure: A Woman's Guide to Getting the Sex You Want, Need, and Deserve.* London: Penguin Books, 2006.

Kavaler, Elizabeth, M.D. *A Seat on the Aisle, Please!* New York: Copernicus Books, 2006.

Moldwin, Robert, M.D. *The Interstitial Cystitis Survival Guide.* Oakland, Calif.: New Harbinger Publications, 2000.

Northrup, Christiane. *The Wisdom of Menopause.* New York: Bantam, 2001.

Stewart, Elizabeth G, M.D. *The V Book: A Doctor's Guide to Complete Vulvovaginal Health.* New York: Bantam, 2002.

Whipple, Beverly, John D. Perry, and Alice Khan Ladas. *The G Spot and Other Discoveries About Human Sexuality.* New York: Bantam, 1982.

Wise, David, Ph.D., and Rodney Anderson, M.D. *A Headache in the Pelvis: A New Understanding and Treatment for Prostatitis and Chronic Pelvic Pain Syndromes.* Occidental, Calif.: National Center for Pelvic Pain Research, 2006.

WHAT PATIENTS SAY

If you suffer from pelvic floor disorder, there are two essential truths to keep in mind always: First, you are not alone. Second, there is help and hope for an end to your pain and discomfort.

Here's the evidence for those truths: testimonials, in their own words, from people who have suffered the very dysfunction from which you are suffering. As you will see, these are men, women, and children, ranging in age from 4 to 75, who have experienced a range of disorders and conditions from chronic holding pattern to post–prostate cancer pain to a bad fall to inflammatory conditions, and more. Some improved quickly—within three months or less. For others, complete healing took as long as a year. What all of these patients had in common, however, was their dedication to their healing and to the discipline of the natural therapies in this book. They also shared an eagerness to let others—like you—know that it is possible to "get your life back," without medication or surgery, from the pain and suffering of pelvic floor disorder. I'm grateful to them, and I know you will be too.

Six months after a laparotomy due to endometriosis, the doctor wanted to send me for surgery again. Another doctor told me that the pain could be due to scar tissue from surgery. Not wanting surgery after surgery, I looked for other alternatives. I started working with a nutritionist and with Amy Stein at Beyond Basics. Amy uses pelvic floor therapy to alleviate muscle cramping and pain due to endometriosis and tissue massage to help loosen scar tissue. After working with Amy, I no longer am in constant pain but have finally gained back feeling and mobility in my abdominal area. She also taught me stretching exercises to do during the week. When I feel pain coming on, which is not often anymore, instead of reaching for aspirin or running back to the doctor, I do these exercises. I feel like I have my life back, I never went back for another surgery and my jumbo size bottles of Advil, Tylenol, and Tylenol PM have expired.

—Kimberly Perez

About seven years ago I was coping with a major physical problem, dysuria or extreme pain when urinating—and for hours thereafter. I had consulted several urologists, and they all had the same diagnosis: chronic prostatitis or bladder infection. The treatment was always the same, too: antibiotics, Flomax, and pain medication. I never got relief, and as a matter of fact the problem was getting worse.

I was watching a public access television program one evening and I heard a very bright M.D. describe pelvic floor disorders as well as interstitial cystitis. I thought to myself, that's it, that's my problem. I promptly made an appointment with a doctor who, after testing me for interstitial cystitis—it was negative—informed me that I had pelvic floor muscle disorder and referred me to Amy Stein.

I met with Amy, who made an assessment and started me on a program of stretching and manipulation. Most importantly, she educated me as to pelvic floor issues, their causes, and treatments.

After three or four months I was 80 percent to 90 percent better, the frequent painful urinations were virtually gone, and I had an awareness of the pelvic floor musculature and could help alleviate my symptoms by stretching and limiting aggravating activities.

Having worked through this problem, I understand the feelings of isolation and hopelessness.

There is hope and help.

—Patrick Appello, 53

I have had severe endometriosis for many years and have had several surgeries. I also started having another type of pain, which was very severe. It felt to me like bladder spasms, and I was having frequent urination every 20 minutes all day long. I finally went to an excellent urologist who was able to feel my pelvic floor muscles through an internal exam and found that my pelvic floor muscles were in spasm (or hypertonic). He prescribed Ativan for a very short term and physical therapy. It seems that after years of pain in my abdomen, I had clenched my abdominal and pelvic floor muscles so much that they were in a constant holding or tightening pattern and they had lost their normal function.

My physical therapist was able to help me through massage techniques and reeducation of the muscles, and with exercises that I could do at home. Finally I began to feel normal again. I am so thankful!!

—Dale Staunton

I was recommended to Amy for an unrelenting problem of burning in my urethra and a "conflict" between my bladder and bowel, when either was full. These problems were brought about by a seed implant therapy performed to cure my prostate cancer. The cancer was cured, but the issues described continued.

Amy did a thorough debriefing of all the issues and went back into my medical history. At the end of the assessment, she advised me that I had pelvic floor muscle tightness in addition to weakness; she was confident, based on her previous treatment of the issues I described, that she would be successful, and indeed after a period of time, the issues were resolved. Physical therapy treatment, as well as my daily home program, consisted of massage techniques, stretching, cardiovascular exercise, and relaxation techniques, specifically those for the pelvic floor. Once my symptoms calmed down, we eventually moved on to core strengthening and I went back to my weight training at the gym.

—Don Friedman, 75

Five years ago, I started experiencing urgency and frequency of urination. Every blood test and examination came out fine. I was told numerous times that there was nothing wrong with me. But I knew something was terribly wrong. As more symptoms started to progress, I became more persistent with the medical professionals. I began having horrible stomach attacks, pain during sexual intercourse, and I was running to the bathroom every 20 minutes to empty my bladder. Sometimes I felt such a strong urge to urinate but actually did not have to go at all. I was waking up five to seven times every night to use the bathroom. I wasn't getting any sleep and could barely eat anything without having a stomach attack. I also started having severe lower back pain. My whole life was thrown upside down.

I was finally diagnosed with interstitial cystitis, a chronic painful bladder disease. Basically, I had no lining around my bladder, which caused the stomach attacks, usually from alcohol or foods that were acidic. I was convinced to have a very painful surgical procedure done called cystoscopy with hydrodistension. I was told this procedure would relieve some of my symptoms, but it only made them worse. After being diagnosed, I was prescribed several different medications—such as 600 mg of Elmiron to help repair the bladder lining and reduce my frequency and urgency of urination, Tigan for nausea caused by the Elmiron, hydrocodone and Lortab for pain associated with my stomach attacks and pain during sexual intercourse, hydroxyzine to help me sleep through the night, and Prevacid for gastritis caused by all of the other medications. I felt like a walking pharmacy.

The Interstitial Cystitis Association recommended that I see a doctor in New York. He examined me and immediately lowered my dosage of Elmiron, stating that the amount I was on was for a 300-pound man when I was a 125-pound woman. This physician diagnosed me with pelvic floor dysfunction and surprisingly did not prescribe me more medication; instead he urged me to see Amy Stein, a physical therapist specializing in pelvic floor dysfunction.

At first, I was confused. I could not understand how a physical therapist could help with my increasingly painful and uncomfortable symptoms of the bladder. At this point, I was so desperate to get my life back, I was willing to try anything. I started seeing Amy in 2002. I lived about two hours from her office. Amy wanted me to come three times a week because my symptoms were so bad, but I could not do this. So, Amy insisted that I come at least once a week. The sessions were painful at first. My pelvic floor muscles were so spasmed and weak. But when I went home, I felt so much better. Amy gave me exercises and relaxation techniques to do at home to relax my spasmed pelvic floor muscles. It was a lot of work but worth it. Physical therapy is not a quick fix. It is a long process but it works. Now, I've been weaned off *all* of the medication.

If I feel a bladder or pelvic floor attack coming on, I will practice my deep breathing or exercises I learned from physical therapy. I have been off all medication for over a year and a half now. I sleep through the night, rarely ever waking up in the middle of the night to go the bathroom. Physical therapy has taught me to retrain my bladder, strengthen my core muscles, and learn to relax my pelvic floor muscles instead of tightening them. Instead of numbing my pain with medication, physical therapy has fixed my pain. Today, I have little pain and limited urgency and frequency of urination. I know how to deal with my pain and discomfort now. Physical therapy has given me my life back. My pelvic floor muscles are so much stronger, which causes less pain and less frequency and urgency of urination. It was definitely a long process, but I have made so much progress and am living my normal life again.

—Jaime McCarty, 29, currently expecting her first child

I had a propensity for bladder frequency all my life as well as sensitivity to myriad of foods and medications. Finally, what was called "urethral syndrome" was given a scientific name: interstitial cystitis. I worked through pain and limitations due to infections as well as the knot of pain on the left side of my abdomen and sexual discomfort by reading a lot about my disease and joining self-help groups. Nonetheless, IC has affected every fiber of who am I, which includes claustrophobia if I'm not seated on an aisle seat.

When I was diagnosed with pelvic floor syndrome, Amy Stein was recommended to me. At that time I attended a self-help group where the leader of the group said, "Sure, I know I can lie down on the floor and do exercises but I won't, so I'll just keep taking my meds." I chose "the floor," and a commitment to see Amy regularly for internal treatments.

Amy's pelvic program, diaphragmatic breathing, cognizance of good bladder habits, and spinal-strength and stabilization exercise are my ongoing home treatment commitment to myself. Working at posture, stretching and working out at the gym is my norm. Mostly, Amy's status as my coach remains a priceless mind/body support as I do my best to age graciously and intelligently.

—Joan K. Levine, aging gracefully

On October 15, 2004, my son Joseph, at the age of nine, came to me with a problem. Joseph was not able to hold any food; it was coming up, and whole food was not breaking down. Joseph was not able to make any stool; it would be in him for weeks before he could go to the bathroom. His stomach would swell up.

I took Joseph right to the hospital where they gave him an enema. When that didn't work, they told me to follow up with his pediatrician. I went the next day to the pediatrician who recommended a hospital specialist. This specialist did several tests and gave Joseph MiraLax to start with until the test results came back. Joseph, who had been out of school for over a year, was taking the MiraLax twice a day. When the tests finally came back, the specialist said the issue was Joseph's anal sphincter, but he said the only thing he could recommend was to go to Boston Children's Hospital for bowel surgery. The doctor also said he would soon be attending a conference where he would bring up Joseph's problem; maybe another doctor would have a solution.

I then got a phone call from the doctor saying that Amy Stein in New York City might be able to help Joseph with his problem because of her experience with biofeedback and pelvic floor dysfunction. I went to New York to meet with Amy to see if she could help. She did. I thank her so much for taking this on because I did not know where to turn next. Amy has helped my son so much, and I am so happy that my son is back in school now and was able to avoid surgery. Amy got him to eat food high in fiber and to be more relaxed so he does not tighten up when he goes to make stool. She also has him doing several exercises that help Joseph. I am so happy to say that Joseph has been off MiraLax for two and half years already thanks to Amy. This has been a wonderful outcome for my son.

—Fulgencia Roberts, Joseph's mother

I began having unbearable bladder problems such as burning, frequency, urgency, pain, and swelling that would sometimes leave me desperate and depressed. I also suffered from severe lower back and hip pain although my MRI was negative for any back dysfunction. I was told I might have interstitial cystitis (a bladder disorder) and there wasn't much to do for this. After many doctor visits and many "dismissals" as if I was making up my symptoms, a nurse practitioner suggested I try pelvic floor therapy. I was lucky enough to find Amy through an Internet search. I was a bit skeptical at first, but three months into treatment I had my life back. Three years later, I continue to keep up with the massage techniques and pelvic floor relaxation exercises. I am eternally grateful for Amy and her treatment and knowledge.

—Carla Szulman, 42

In 1995, at the age of 24, after seeing eight or nine different gyne-cologists, I was diagnosed by one of them with a condition known as vulvodynia. At that time I had never heard of such a thing. I had suffered with some form of pelvic discomfort since the age of 13. The pain back then was intermittent and only bothered me when I was wearing tight jeans, riding a bike, or walking or sitting for long periods at a time. I had a surgical procedure called a partial vulvectomy in an attempt to relieve the pain. Although the surgery helped relieve some of the local pain in the vaginal area, my overall pelvic pain had become constant and unbearable. I was prescribed Elavil, which helped me a great deal. I didn't have constant pain any more, but was still unable to have intercourse or any form of penetration even with a tampon. Over time I developed a bad reac-tion to the Elavil and had to stop taking it. My pain returned worse than ever before. I then went to a pain management specialist and a neurologist, but both offered no relief. I tried acupuncture, anti-histamines, antibiotics, antifungal treatments, and a low oxalate diet, but none of that helped at all. A new medication called Neu-rontin came on the market, but offered me only limited relief. At this point, now 32, I was happily married for two years; however, I was still unable to tolerate any penetration, and therefore, unable to have intercourse with my husband.

Then I finally saw a doctor who explained that I had not only vulvodynia, but primary vulvodynia, which means my condition is congenital, not caused by any injury, which would then be called secondary vulvodynia. He also said due to many years of suffering, I had the worst pelvic floor dysfunction he had ever seen. He put me on a medication called Cymbalta to help calm the nerve pain and referred me to Beyond Basics for physical therapy to correct the pelvic floor dysfunction. Within just weeks and after a few minor setbacks, I was better overall than I had been in my life. I attended weekly therapy visits, performed daily exercises, and worked at home with a dilator as well as doing deep breathing exercises and various massage techniques. I live many days either pain-free or with minimal discomfort, and I have even been able to have intercourse finally with my husband. The symptoms that began at age 13 finally subsided after one year of physical therapy treatment at age 35.

—Christa Kozoriz, 35

Amy Stein's therapies gave me back my life. I experienced a three-month block and then a six-month block of chronic pain and urgency. It was relentless. Having gone to several different doctors, having had every kind of invasive test, having tried all kinds of medicines, even self-catheterization, I felt no relief. Finally I was directed to Amy, and after my very first session I felt almost total relief. I am now better than even before having the problem.

Miracles do happen. This is not by chance. It is by the very clear and sensitive work done by Amy. She teaches you exercises that include both breathing and stretching that you do at home. So she gives you your own tools to both alleviate the problem if you begin sensing the beginnings of it again, and also as a preventative. The internal work is a key element for many sufferers.

—Marika Brown, 49

Our son Milo had trouble going to the toilet as soon as he was out of diapers. We thought he was a bit slow in potty training, but at four, he still had a lot of "accidents." We saw a gastroenterologist for over a year, but the drugs did not work. At the same time, all the exams showed that he had no physiological issues. So we started the physical therapy massages, stretching exercises, and biofeedback. It has helped Milo be more aware of his body, to relax, and to stop holding his stools. We have learned to help with the massages and stretching at home. Milo's condition has improved steadily, without the side effects of drugs. He is now five and a half, and after only four months of therapy, he has no more accidents at school, which is a big relief.

—Milo's parents

I am a professional stock trader. I believe years of straining and reading the *Wall Street Journal* in the bathroom (along with intermittent bouts of hemorrhoids) was more than my pelvic floor could bear. In June 2003, the sell-off in my pelvis started. In a hurry to get on the racquetball court, I strained hard resulting in a sharp pain in the right side of my rectum along with what felt like a firecracker exploding in my left testicle. The pain dissipated in a minute or two. Over the ensuing two to three months I noticed mild intermittent rectal pain, bleeding, and some bowel urgency.

My diagnosis? I had latent trigger points in the rectum, levator, and operator internus activated by anal fissure and fistula. This explains the referred pain pattern in the genitals, rectum, abdomen, back, buttocks, and thighs. The rectal pain was occasionally severe but mostly moderate with an unrelenting quality affecting other parts of the anatomy, making it all the more worse. Specifically, 20 to 30 minutes before a bowel movement, I would feel burning or blunt penis pain, thigh burning, rectal heaviness, low back pain, sometimes all of the above, sometimes a subset. After the bowel movement, the same pain would continue, and on many occasions I literally felt the need to urinate almost constantly for one to two hours. There were some mornings I could not get out of the house without two to three bowel movements; in addition I was now driving to work with a Tupperware container in my car for fear that I would have to urinate. I was also in a panic.

After appointments with two colorectal surgeons, two gastroenterologists, two general practitioners, two urologists, and one osteopath in addition to several anoscopes, a CT scan, two MRIs, and one GI series, the test results all came up negative—except for revealing an anal fissure and fistula. But none of the doctors believed I could experience all this referred pain and urinary urgency/frequency from a fissure and fistula. All but the osteopath! He understood pelvic floor disease and sent me into physical therapy.

I dedicated myself to the exercise programs, massage, relaxation, stretching, nutrition—all the natural therapies Amy prescribes. Thanks to these therapies, I quickly got back to 70 percent of my predisorder state and began to see some light at the end of the tunnel. I even ventured back out onto the racquetball court. Still, I couldn't get back to 100 percent, and Amy and my doctor suggested it was because of the fistula; as a result, it had to be surgically treated.

Back to the natural healing therapies. The pain grew less frequent and less intense. Now, I am 100 percent pain-free and 100 percent cured. I can say my pelvic floor has become a bull market again.

—Mike C., 43

I had a severe case of pelvic floor dysfunction with abdominal, hip, and back pain, and I had trouble with everyday activities like sitting, standing, working, driving, and sexual intercourse. I was finally diagnosed and referred for physical therapy. I was on several medications to help me with the pain, but I wanted to get off them to have children.

I traveled once a week into the city, which took me over an hour. Because my symptoms were so severe, it took several months to gradually get off the meds. Fortunately, my symptoms were improving with each passing month. I took five medications in all: Elmiron, Pyridium Plus, lorazepam, and other pain blocker meds. Once I was off the medications, I conceived pretty quickly.

I continued my PT treatments once a week up into my third trimester. Along with these treatments, my therapist devised an exercise program for me to do at home. It let me keep my muscles intact through the pregnancy. They definitely helped! After giving birth, my symptoms are 90 percent improved. I am told that it's because the muscles are stretched out, which decreases the muscle spasms.

I have mild flare-ups here and there, but I have not been in for a treatment since the birth of my little gemstone, Alexander. I attribute this to the physical therapy and my home exercise program. And, now I have a second child, Clayton. Without my physical therapist's services I would not have my two sons! I have Amy to thank.

—Kristina Kozak, 37

REFERENCES

CHAPTER 3

Fitzgerald, M. P., and R. Kotarinos. "Rehabilitation of the Short Pelvic Floor. II: Treatment of the Patient with the Short Pelvic Floor." *Int Urogynecol J* 14, no. 4 (2003): 269–275.

Wise, D., and R. Anderson. *A Headache in the Pelvis*, 4th ed. Occidental, CA: National Center for Pelvic Pain Research, 2006.

CHAPTER 5

Travell, J., and D. Simons, *The Trigger Point Manual*, vol. 1 (Baltimore, MD: Williams and Wilkins, 1983).

Travell, J., and D. Simons, *The Trigger Point Manual*, vol. 2 (Baltimore, MD: Williams and Wilkins; 1992).

Weiss, J., Prendergast, S. "Screening for Musculoskeletal Causes of Pelvic Pain." *Clinical Obstetrics and Gynecology* 46 (2003): 773-782.

Weiss, Jerome. "Pelvic floor myofascial trigger points: manual therapy for interstitial cystitis and the urgency-frequency syndrome." *J Urol* 166 (2001): 2226-31.

CHAPTER 8

Anderson et al. "Sexual Dysfunction in Men with Chronic Prostatitis/Chronic Pelvic Pain Syndrome: Improvement after Trigger Point Release and Paradoxical Relaxation Training." *J Urol*, Oct 2005, 1534–38.

Darbre, P. D., A. Aljarrah, W. R. Miller, N. G. Coldham, M. J. Sauer, and G. S. Pope. "Concentrations of Parabens in Human Breast Tumours." *J Appl Toxicol* 24, no. 1 (Jan–Feb 2004): 5–13.

Golden, Robert, Jay Gandy, and Guenter Vollmer. "A Review of the Endocrine Activity of Parabens and Implications for Potential Risks to Human Health." *Critical Reviews in Toxicology* 35, no. 5 (2005): 435–458.

Harvey, Philip W., and Philippa Darbre. "Endocrine Disrupters and Human Health: Could Estrogenic Chemicals in Body Care Cosmetics Adversely Affect Breast Cancer Incidence in Women? A Review of Evidence and Call for Further Research." *Journal of Applied Toxicology* 24, no. 3 (2004): 167–176.

Nickel, J. C., et al. "Prevalence of Prostatitis-Like Symptoms in a Population Based Study Using the National Institutes of Health Chronic Prostatitis Symptom Index." *J Urol* 165 (2001): 842.

Perry, John Delbert, and Beverly Whipple. The Varieties of Female Orgasm and Female Ejaculation." *SIECUS Report* IX, no. 5/6 (May–July 1981).

CHAPTER 9

Borg-Stein, Joanne, et al. "Musculoskeletal Aspects of Pregnancy." *Am J Phys Med Rehabil* 84, no. 3 (2005): 180–192.

Wurn, Belinda, et al. "Treating Female Infertility and Improving IVF Pregnancy Rates with a Manual Physical Therapy Technique." *Med Gen Med* 6 (2) (2004): 1–17.

CHAPTER 11

Anderson R., et al. "Integration of Myofascial Trigger Point Release and Paradoxical Relaxation Training Treatment of Chronic Pelvic Pain in Men." *J Urol* 174 (2005): 155–160. 2005.

Anderson, R. U., et al. "Sexual Dysfunction in Men with Chronic Prostatitis/Chronic Pelvic Pain Syndrome: Improvement After Trigger Point Release and Paradoxical Relaxation Training." *J Urol* 176 (Oct 2006): 1534–8.

Barbalias, G. A., et al. "Prostatodynia: Clinical and Urodynamic Characteristics." *J Urol* 130 (1983): 514.

Hetrick, D. C., et al. "Musculoskeletal Dysfunction in Men with Chronic Pelvic Pain Syndrome Type III: A Case-Study." *J Urol* 170 (2003): 828.

Nickel, J. C., et al. "Prevalence of Prostatitis-Like Symptoms in a Population Based Study Using the National Institutes of Health Chronic Prostatitis Symptom Index." *J Urol* 165 (2001): 842.

APPENDIX A

Fitzgerald, M. P., and R. Kotarinos, "Rehabilitation of the Short Pelvic Floor. I: Background and Patient Evaluation," *International Urogynecol J* 14 (2003): 261–268.

Howard, F. M., Perry, C. P., Carter, J. E., et al. "Pelvic Pain Diagnosis and Management." Philadelphia: Lippincott Williams & Wilkins, 2000.

Steege, J. F., Metzger, D. A., Levy B. *Chronic Pelvic Pain: An Integrated Approach*. Philadelphia: W. B. Saunders Company, 1998.

Travell, J., and D. Simons, *The Trigger Point Manual*, vol. 1 (Baltimore, MD: Williams and Wilkins, 1983).

Travell, J., and D. Simons, *The Trigger Point Manual*, vol. 2 (Baltimore, MD: Williams and Wilkins; 1992).

Weiss, Jerome M., "Chronic Pelvic Pain and Myofascial Trigger Points," *The Pain Clinic* 2, no. 6 (December 2000): 13–18.

INDEX